Advance Praise

Intimate and vulnerably transparent, Robert Rickelman's memoir invites readers into the unvarnished experience of living with and around mental illness and alcoholism. Unflinchingly candid, the author resists easy explanations or tidy conclusions, offering instead a lived narrative that is both painful and deeply human.

—Natalia Loya Herrera, Author of *The Laboratory Assistant*

Robert Rickelman's *Jumping to the End* is a gripping, courageous, and compulsively readable memoir that tells the truth about one man's journey to rock bottom, and back. Robert's extraordinary storytelling manages to be both heartbreaking and heart-opening as he narrates his powerful experiences trying to survive law school with the aid of alcohol, plunging ever deeper into alcoholism and mental illness. Robert's memoir is a love letter penned from the abyss, never shying away from the darkest parts of the human condition, while also illuminating the friendship, connection, and love that can be found on even the most painful journeys through life. A healing and hopeful must-read for those whose family trees are haunted by addiction and secrecy.

—Summer Dawn Hammond, author of *The Impossible Why*

Jumping to the End is a window into an unspoken world of perseverance despite deep despair in the midst of addiction. It is an inspiring tale of a man with severe mental illness striving to find normalcy—a story of inspiration and resilience, losses and gains.

—Dylan Williams, High-school English Teacher

JUMPING TO THE END

JUMPING TO THE END

A Lifetime Struggle with Mental Illness and Alcoholism

A Memoir

Robert Rickelman

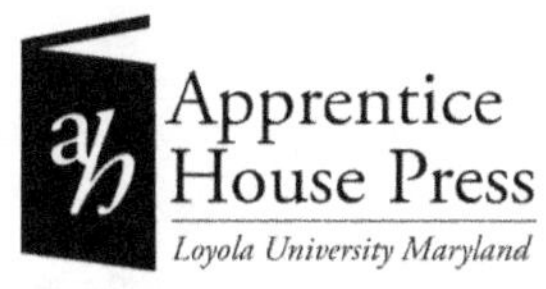

First Edition

Casebound ISBN: 978-1-62720-659-4
Paperback ISBN: 978-1-62720-660-0
Ebook ISBN: 978-1-62720-661-7

Design by Caroline Corr
Editorial Development by Samantha Vitale
Promotional Development by Ashley Lopez

Published by Apprentice House Press

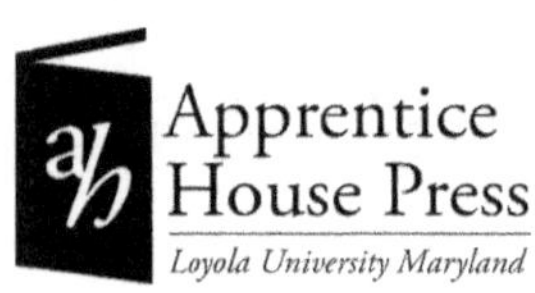

Loyola University Maryland
4501 N. Charles Street, Baltimore, MD 21210
410.617.5265
www.ApprenticeHouse.com
info@ApprenticeHouse.com

Contents

Contents

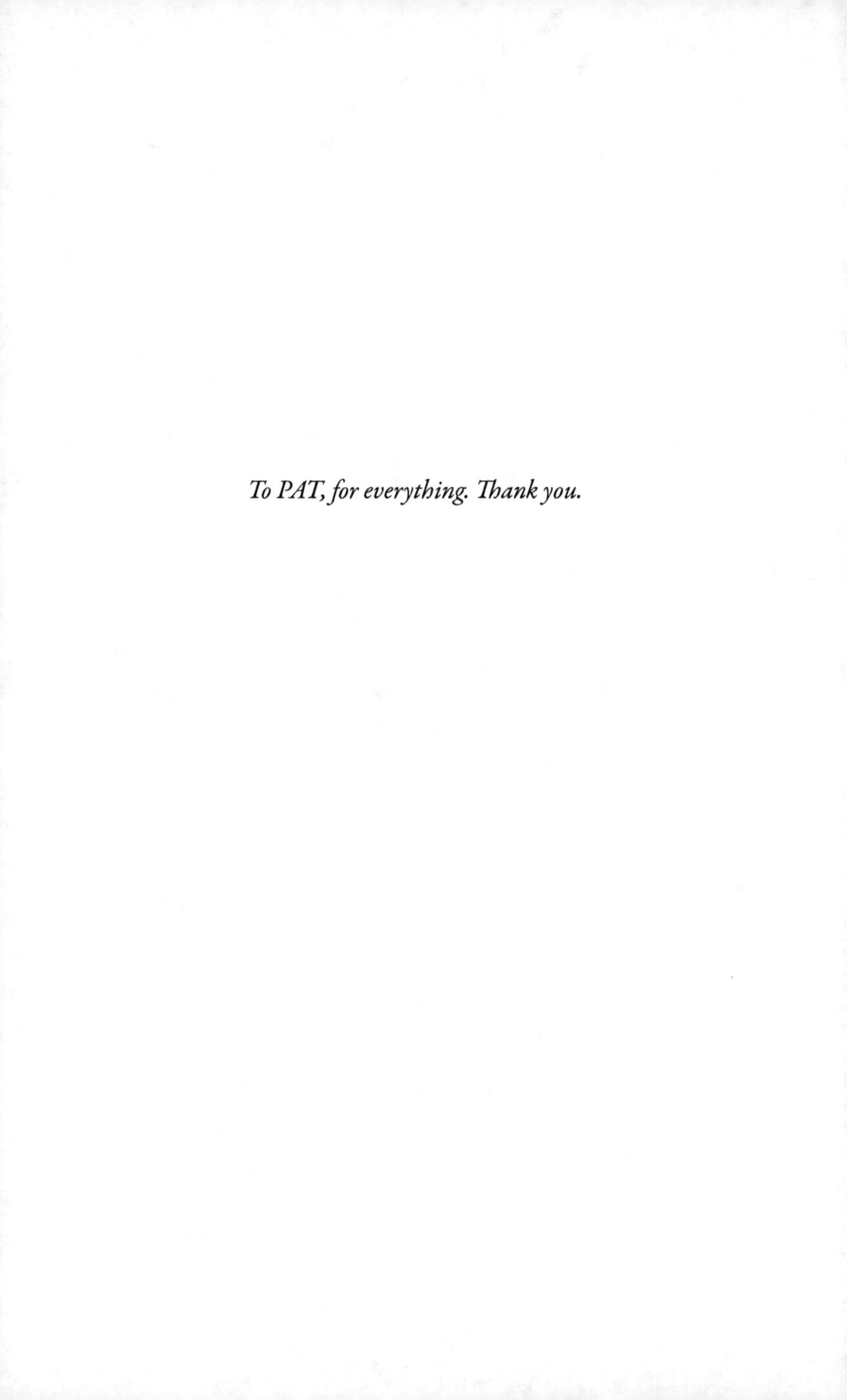

To PAT, for everything. Thank you.

Acknowledgments

I'd like to acknowledge the following publications in which several of my stories originally appeared; some were differently titled or in slightly different form: "Phyllis," (*Inscape Magazine*); "Group Therapy," (*Twisted Vine Literary Arts Journal*); "Orange Sweater" and "Comic Relief," (*The Long Island Literary Journal)*; "Leaving Prince Albert," (*Blue River Review*); "Awake in the ICU," (*Barely South Review*); "Anniversary Flowers," (*Adelaide Magazine*); "ACHIEVE," (*Dual Coast Magazine*); "Psychokinesis," (*Nixes Mate Review*); and "13th and Island Detox." (*Panoply, A Literary Zine*).

Preface

In Matthew 6:34, Jesus says, "So never be anxious about the next day, for the next day will have its own anxieties. Each day has enough of its own troubles." Wise counsel, but here's my take: today will suck and so will tomorrow and the next day. My wife, Pat, tells me, "You never live in the moment; you always want to jump to the end." She's right, I want to get everything over with as quickly as possible. And this is why—I'm afraid of looking stupid. Almost every social interaction is torture, and my goal is to end every conversation without making a fool of myself. If I can manage to finish with something clever, so much the better. But the bottom line is, I don't want anything hanging over my head. I want no unfinished business to dread.

CHAPTER 1

Awake in the ICU

I came to. Rather, I had a vague awareness that I was still alive. My mind was swimming. A played-out metaphor, if not for the fact that my brain and body had been bombarded by booze for the last 30 years. I was in a hospital, probably the ICU. That was the drill whenever I mixed my psych meds and alcohol. I thought I'd ingested enough of everything to do the trick this time, but there I was again, alive and breathing. My throat burned raw from the friction of the ventilator tube that had saved my life. I hated being intubated. But then again, I hated a lot of things. Most of all, I hated being alive.

I felt a soft hand gently stroking my tangled hair. Something wet—a drop—landed on my left arm. It was a tear. Things were coming slowly into view. My wife, Pat, was standing at my side. Her nose was red, her eyes bloodshot and swollen. She dabbed her tears with a crumpled blue tissue. Standing next to her was a pretty, young woman wearing blue scrubs.

"Good morning, Robert. I'm Kirsten, your nurse. It's good to see you awake. I hope you realize how fortunate you are. You had a very close call."

As I grew more alert, the breathing tube felt like a fist had been shoved down my throat. I fought the urge to gag.

"You need to relax, Robert," Kirsten said. "Breathe slowly and deeply. Try not to think about the tube."

I wanted to ask when they were going to remove it, but my voice was barely audible. I motioned for something to write with. Pat reached into her purse for a pen and gave me a folded envelope to write on.

"How much longer for the tube?" I scrawled. My shaky writing made scarcely more sense than my labored whispers.

"Now that you're conscious," Kirsten said, "we'll watch you for a few hours, and if everything's okay, we'll remove the tube. You're going to be with us for a few more days."

Not what I'd wanted to hear, but I had no one to blame but myself.

Another source of discomfort was the catheter for my bladder, which stung whenever I moved. I hoped that the nurse would be removing it soon. That was going to smart.

I wanted to know what day it was. I scribbled another question.

"It's Wednesday morning, February 5. They brought you here Monday afternoon," Pat said. She began to weep.

"I came home and found you passed out in the bathtub. You still had your shoes on. And the wastebasket . . . it was on fire. You could have been killed," she sobbed. "You could have burned our house down!"

I had put Pat through a terrifying ordeal.

"You are one lucky man," the nurse repeated.

I didn't feel lucky. Not lucky at all.

CHAPTER 2

Crybaby

I've been fucked up since I was a kid. My first memories are of an intense and overwhelming shyness, which made me an easy target of teasing and downright bullying. My refuge was our backyard swing set, where I'd soar through the air, safe and secure in my isolation. I was a crybaby, but I was not a tattletale. This didn't speak to a strong moral fiber; I simply realized that tattling would invite additional torment.

I was afraid of everything. Well, technically, I wasn't afraid of my own shadow, but since it was a projection of me, I didn't much care for it either.

CHAPTER 3

Orange Sweater

I first grasped the severity of my mom's alcoholism when I was seven years old. Whenever we would have a party at our house—say for Thanksgiving, Christmas, Holy Communion, or whatever—my mom would get blotto and would take to her bed the following day, staying drunk for at least a week, often longer. This pattern rarely changed. Any time there was a party, Mom would go on a binge.

And her drinking only got worse. Often her sprees would start when she and my dad went out to dinner, which always involved too many martinis, and devolved into an argument about Mom's overdoing it—again.

At least once or twice a month, my mother's Aunt Eleanor (my Grandpa's sister), perhaps not quite a lush herself, but a heavy drinker, would drop by on a weekday afternoon, when we all knew my dad, a full-fledged workaholic attorney, would not be home for hours.

Aunt Eleanor would arrive, armed with four quarts of Drewerys Beer, which she and my mom would share. When the beer was gone, she'd be on her merry way. Then I'd watch as my mother stashed the empties deep inside the garbage can in the alley, and brushed her teeth two, maybe three times, before my father arrived home, usually at 7:30.

Back then, I thought the brushing must have worked because, as my mother served the dinner that she always kept warm for him, my father never questioned her about her breath. Now, looking back and learning firsthand that brushing your teeth does not mask booze breath, I think he just resigned himself to her drinking. And besides, when my mom drank, my dad had the freedom to do what he wanted. He could work late, and my mom wouldn't complain as long as she could knock down some beers while he was away.

When my mom's binges went on too long, the mountains of dirty laundry reached considerable heights. When I was nine or ten, I was getting good grades at school, and my father reasoned that of all the older kids, I would be the one least affected by missing school, so I was tasked with staying home and restoring the house to order. I have to agree that I was the best candidate for the job, and I kind of liked skipping out on school and having the house to myself while my mom remained in her soporific state. The work was hard and tedious, but I did get to watch my TV game shows all day long. I never watched soap operas. I hated them. Besides, my life was its own telenovela.

By this time, my father was making a very good living, and we were able to afford two washers and two dryers. Still, doing so much laundry was a daunting responsibility. Also, the young ones had to eat, and there were school lunches to pack, dishes to do, and a large house to clean. At nine or ten, I was old enough to recognize when my mom's drinking had settled into its final, most desperate stage, and I would worry about her.

As I said, none of this was affecting my grades. I was a student at Sacred Heart School, back in the days when the nuns could still take their swats at any pint-sized miscreants. I generally stayed out of trouble and out of their reach.

After a few days of my staying home, I think that guilt and shame would overcome my mother, or her money would run out, and she'd stop drinking. When she was drunk, she always wore this ratty old, orangish-gold sweater. I loathed that sweater. But, of all the kids, the one who should have hated that fucking sweater the most was my brother Kurt, who had the misfortune of being born on New Year's Day.

Every New Year, my grandparents would arrive, my grandmother would bake a cake, and the family would gather in the kitchen to sing "Happy Birthday" to Kurt. And every time we gathered, my mother would stumble out of her bedroom, wearing that god-damned fucking sweater, and she'd parrot the same worn-out pledge to Kurt. "I promise next year will be different," she'd slur. "I'll be better for your next birthday. I will." God, how I wanted to burn that fucking sweater and all the wretchedness it possessed.

When my mom finally started to sober up, I'd feel so sorry for her. I loved her, and I knew she was ashamed of what she was doing. She just couldn't help herself. One drink and she couldn't stop. So, when the drinking ceased, I'd bring her some soft-boiled eggs, dry toast, and glasses of 7-Up to nurse her back to health.

It was tough to watch as she struggled to steady her trembling hands and take a bite of food or a sip of soda. There were many times when she couldn't keep anything down, and I'd bring her a bowl to vomit into or help her to the bathroom to throw up. God, how I loved that poor, sick woman. Nowadays, I guess you'd refer to her drinking as "self-medicating," but back then, it was the only way she could deal with the demons that raged within.

CHAPTER 4

Coralee

My final semester at the University of Illinois had drawn to a close. It was mid-May of 1977, and I would soon embark on what I hoped would be a successful three years at John Marshall Law School in Chicago. My father had arranged to drive down to Urbana and bring me home. Simple enough—or so I thought.

My dad arrived on a Saturday morning with a guest in tow. And he was about to drop a bombshell. The doorbell rang. It was him, and he was wearing an uncharacteristically sheepish expression. He hugged me, always an uncomfortable moment.

"Hi, Dad. How was the ride down?" I asked.

"Um, Rob, I've brought someone I want you to meet."

This is probably the last thing a kid wants to hear from a parent. I felt a wave of nausea.

Oh fucking shit, I know what he's going to say. You motherfucking asshole. Don't fucking say it.

"Down here?" I stumbled for words. "In Urbana?"

"Rob, you know that your mother and I have not been close for the last several years. I've met someone, and she's very nice. She's waiting in the car. I'd really like you to meet her. Get to know her."

And I'd really like you to go fuck yourself.

"Wow, Dad, this is so unexpected. I don't know what to say."

"Well, Rob, she's in the car, and we all need to get back to Chicago. What do you say? She's more anxious than you are."

"I don't know about that."

"Please, Rob . . . do this . . . do it for me."

I didn't know what to say. How in the fuck could he do this to me? To my mom? What kind of snake would I be if I gave in to this "meet my new friend" horseshit? I was flummoxed. Flummoxed and fucked.

I grabbed some things and made my way to the car. I was expecting his flashy, 1975 burgundy Buick Electra with its matching vinyl top. The Electra was the first car he had bought since our 1960 Ford Falcon that wasn't a station wagon. I should have noticed then, the subtle change in my father's character when he decided to abandon the family-man image in favor of the Buick "Deuce-and-a-Quarter." My mom had wanted another station wagon, but she didn't drive, and my dad always got his way.

I walked to the street and was struck by a beautiful, brand-new, dark-brown, 1977 Cadillac Fleetwood. It was a car that made the statement, "Look at me. I've arrived." The Fleetwood was fully loaded and had gorgeous tan leather seats. My father never bought used cars, and our family had come to expect a new car every other year. Once again, my father did not disappoint.

It was nearly noon. I spotted a blonde-haired woman sitting in the front passenger seat. I hesitated.

My father was directly behind me when I stopped.

"Rob, her name is Coralee. I'm sure you'll like her. Do this for me."

"Do this for you," I thought. *"You selfish fucking bastard!"*

"God, Dad, this is so uncomfortable."

"C'mon, just let's meet her."

As we reached the car, he opened the door, and Coralee

stepped out. He never opened the door for my mom, the bastard.

"Hi," she chirped with an annoying southern accent. "You must be Rob." She offered her hand. "I'm Coralee, Coralee Edwards, and I'm pleased to make your acquaintance."

And I'm Rob, the weasel who's about to stick a knife in his mother's back.

She was a brassy blonde, probably in her late thirties, at least fifteen years younger than he was. And her breasts. She had very large breasts. I've never liked big boobs, but I guessed that's what he found attractive about her.

"Hi," I said. I shook her hand.

"Well, I guess I don't need to tell you how much you resemble your father. How many girlfriends you have is what I'd like to know."

Give me a fucking break.

"I'm not much of a ladies' man," I said.

"Oh, I reckon you do just fine with the ladies. I have a sixth sense about these things."

"Not to change the subject," I said, "but I detect a southern twang. Where are you from, Coralee?"

"I was born and raised in Montgomery, Alabama. I graduated from the University of Alabama in 1967 with a degree in business. 'Roll Tide.' I got married that same year, and my husband and I settled in Birmingham. We divorced in 1975, and I moved to Chicago. I settled into my condo on North Kenilworth in Oak Park, and I still live there today. Now, I'm a loan officer at First National Bank of Chicago. I work downtown, and I just love my job."

"Sounds great," I said. I had nothing left to say and went back to collect the rest of my things.

After I had loaded the car, we were ready to go. It was going to be a long drive home.

"Well," my father said, "why don't we stop for lunch before we get on the highway? What's a good place for lunch, Rob?"

"Um, Boar's Head Inn," I blurted out before I remembered that this was the restaurant where my mom, dad, uncle, and aunt had shared a meal one homecoming weekend a few years earlier. The nausea returned.

"Sounds good," he said. "They open for lunch?"

"Pretty sure," I said.

We found the restaurant, and, once again, my father gallantly opened the door for his lady friend. I cringed. I spent the better part of that day cringing and feeling sick to my stomach.

Coralee talked a mile a minute, and it was obvious that she was mighty proud to be dating a lawyer. Well, my mom was married to a lawyer, and where did that get her? I barely touched my food, but I did polish off three vodka tonics—all doubles.

Finally, we reached Oak Park and dropped off Coralee at her condo. When we got home, my mom gave me a big hug. I hugged her back, real hard. I wanted to fucking cry.

CHAPTER 5

Emma

While spending the summer getting a feel for the practice of law at my dad's firm, I decided it would be a good idea to enroll in an evening class of accounting at Triton College, which was a fairly large junior college about two miles from home. My younger brother, Kurt, usually gave me a ride to and from school in my father's fancy Fleetwood.

There were about 40 students in the class. The instructor was a very good-natured woman of about 40. Her name was Ms. Hammond; she never told us her first name. She had an easy-going way about her, and her love of the subject matter was obvious and infectious.

We were still in late June, and I wouldn't be starting law school until the end of August. But the days were passing rapidly. I would be a law student in no time. Was I ready? As far as the academic rigors of law school, I was confident, but I wasn't sure I was prepared for the performance aspect that was a large part of attending law school. I never shared this self-doubt with a soul. No one could be privy to this closely guarded secret.

Among my accounting classmates was a girl, pretty but not a knockout, who exuded such poise and elegance that I was immediately drawn to her. Her name was Emma Sloan, and her father was a successful doctor. She was about to enter her final year at Georgetown University. She was majoring in English with a minor in Art History, and she had not yet decided whether to work toward a doctorate in English or attend law school. She was very bright, and I did not doubt that she would excel in any field she chose.

As it turned out, I wasn't the only student who was taken by Emma's charm. The other guy was Frank Carlini. He was an Italian from Cicero, a blue-collar town that borders Chicago's southwest side. It's where Al Capone moved his operation after being forced out of Chicago. Cicero was mostly working-class white, with many Czechs and Italians.

Frank claimed to own a small used-car lot, but for some reason, he frequently caught a ride home with Kurt and me. He showed us pictures of his business with a sign declaring "Carlini Motors: Fine Used Cars, Great Low Prices." The pictures were pretty convincing, so we didn't question the veracity of his claim.

Frank was full of machismo, despite being about five foot six or seven, and a bit on the pudgy side. He wore his wiry black hair slicked back and sported long bushy sideburns and the porn-star mustache that was so popular in the late '70s. I, on the other hand, was clean-shaven, and although I was 22 years old, I could easily get away without shaving for several days at a time.

Frank was as enamored of Emma as I was and told both Kurt and me that he was going to ask her out after our final exam. Now, I was no Robert Redford, but Kurt encouraged me by reminding me that I was much better looking and more refined than Frank. But Frank was a salesman, and he was certain he could impress Emma.

Before long, it was time for finals. Both Frank and I were preparing our strategies for landing a date with the enchanting Emma. In the meantime, I studied long and hard for the exam, and it paid off.

We took the test on a Thursday evening, and on Tuesday, our last class, Ms. Hammond announced, "Well, everyone, I have evaluated your exams, and I want to tell you that only one student achieved a perfect score. Congratulations, Mr. Rickelman, you earned a 100 percent."

I was floored. I was both flattered and embarrassed to have my score announced to the entire class. Frank did not look happy. He probably realized—correctly—that my 100 percent would be the winning ticket in the Date Emma Sloan Sweepstakes.

After class, I thanked our instructor for teaching us so well. And I genuinely meant it; she was an excellent teacher. Emma joined me in saying thanks and farewell to our gracious instructor.

As for my test score, I wanted Emma to gush. But she didn't. She smiled gracefully and simply said, "One hundred percent. Congratulations, Rob."

"Thanks," I said. "I studied hard every day, so I just had to review the material."

"Nevertheless, you should be proud."

Nevertheless. She could say *"nevertheless,"* and it didn't sound at all affected. I was smitten. I felt bad for Frank, but I knew that I was going to get her to go out with me.

Fortunately, I had driven to class that evening, and I chatted with Emma as we headed to the parking lot. Frank was not around.

"May I walk you to your car?" I asked.

"Thank you, that would be nice."

"So, when do you leave for Georgetown?"

"I leave in two weeks," she answered.

"Would you maybe like to go out to dinner, see a play, or something?"

See a play? See a fucking play, or something? Rob, you fucking nitwit.

She chuckled. "Oh, I don't know. Do you see many plays?"

My ears were burning. They get very red when I'm embarrassed, and boy, was I embarrassed. "Well, not really. But I saw something about *Bleacher Bums* at the Organic Theater."

"It's an interesting title," she said

"I guess. It's about a bunch of diehard Cubs fans. I think it's a comedy."

"So, are you a Cubs fan?"

"Sox fan, but there aren't any plays about them this week."

"Not bad, Rob," I thought.

She smiled. I loved how she smiled. I felt she was growing prettier by the moment. I was getting nervous again.

"I would love to see *Bleacher Bums* with you."

She said yes. Was I up for this? Man, classy girls scared the shit out of me.

"Great, what night is good for you?"

"Well, isn't Saturday night date night?"

She was good at this. Very composed and confident.

"Saturday, yeah, sure. Sounds great. I'll have to check the times. Can I call you?'

She wrote her phone number on my hand. My palms were damp. I hoped her number wouldn't wear off.

"Call me when you find out." She got into her car and smiled.

I returned her smile and turned away. She started the engine and was gone.

Yes, yes, yes. I couldn't wait to tell Kurt. Bad luck for Frank, though.

Emma and I saw *Bleacher Bums* and had a nice dinner afterward. Of course, I had downed a fair amount of vodka before the evening began. I didn't think she noticed. I tried not to breathe too much in her direction, and the date appeared to go well.

The next day, Emma invited me to her house for dinner. I would be meeting her parents. Again, I fortified myself with more vodka. When she introduced me to her mom and dad, I felt they could smell the alcohol on my breath. Thankfully, they served wine with the meal. I was grateful not to have to worry about booze breath, but went easy on the wine, trying to pass myself off as a social drinker. Although I tried mightily to act sober, I think her parents were on to me.

Emma was just days away from returning to Georgetown. We were supposed to go out on the night before she left. On the day before our date, I called to finalize our plans, and she informed me that she had decided to spend her last night in Chicago with some girlfriends. I was crushed. When I got off the phone, I cried. Nobody saw me, but her decision had cut me deeply.

Emma Sloan was the first in a long line of girls who would dump me on account of my drinking. I knew that was why she broke off our date. Although I was upset, I didn't blame her.

Finally, the summer came to a close, and I was prepared to leave the salad days at Farwell, Rickelman, and Proteau. Was I ready? Boy, I wished I knew.

CHAPTER 6

Always Crashing in the Same Car

Finally, it was time to attend registration and orientation at John Marshall Law School. Without knowing much about the organization, I was attracted to the Lawyers Guild. My father explained that it was a communist-affiliated movement, and I might not want to get involved with it.

As it turned out, the school's orientation facilitators emphasized that freshmen would be better served by not engaging in any extracurricular activities. The first-year law students, the facilitators insisted, would have enough on their plates just keeping up with the rigors of law school.

At the start of our first semester, my classmates and I received the designation "J80D3," which meant that we were the afternoon class, scheduled to graduate in June of 1980. "J80D3." I loved the sound of it. It made me feel like an honest-to-god, real-life law student.

My courses that semester were Criminal Law, Torts, Personal Property, Contracts I, and Legal Research and Writing. I took to the academic element of law school fairly easily. It was the classroom experience that would be my undoing.

J80D3 was composed of roughly 130 students. One of the first topics of conversation, a way to size up your classmates, was "What did you get on the LSAT?" I never brought up the subject myself, but I was always eager to answer when a classmate asked me my score. No one in my section had come close to my 696. Even my father, the emotionally detached and very successful trial lawyer, was impressed with my score. His approval was hard to win, but because of the LSAT, he was proud of me.

But a 696 on my LSAT was the only thing I had going for me. Everything else about law school—putting myself out there, speaking in public, being badgered by hostile professors, and shrinking under fire—terrified me.

John Marshall was similar to most law schools in its application of the so-called "Socratic" method of teaching. Most of our professors referred to it more accurately as the adversarial method, where it was a professor's duty to verbally beat you into submission until you were capable of enduring the sorts of harangues you were sure to encounter at the hands of judges in the not-too-distant future.

If it hadn't been so terrifying, it would almost have been laughable to hear the stern voice of the professor as he called on an unlucky student to present his or her case brief, which was then picked to pieces, usually far before the student ever came close to their conclusion. Voices would crack and quiver, hands would tremble, and papers would flutter. But there were a select number of students who lived for the challenge of dueling with the professor. God, how I envied them.

For the most part, we first-year students were scared shitless when our moment in the spotlight arrived. Eventually, though, my fellow students grew accustomed to the routine and delivered their briefs with increasing courage and poise.

Every student but me. I couldn't even respond to a simple follow-up question a professor might lob at me if a student reciting his brief happened to stumble.

I fretted over how I would face the trial by fire that every student was expected to confront. I knew the answer, and it repelled me. My only chance of successfully participating in law school was to drink my way through, and this sad realization shamed me deeply.

Our school day started at 1:00 p.m. and finished at 5:00 p.m., Monday through Friday. It was a schedule remarkably well suited to my habit of studying first, then fortifying myself with the liquid courage I would require to function in the classroom.

Each weekday morning, I would wake at 7:00, and at 8:00, I would pore studiously over my law books, reading my cases and writing my briefs. At 11:00, I'd pour some vodka and orange juice. I needed my screwdrivers. And every morning as I drank, I listened to the same song. It was David Bowie's "Always Crashing in the Same Car." How perfectly that song foreshadowed the calamity that lay ahead.

Our classroom was arranged like an inverted wedding cake. On entering the room, we would see the professor's podium located in the center of a very large semi-circle of long tables arranged in a tiered fashion. In other words, the professor held court from the lowest point of the classroom. Nevertheless, although every student looked down toward the professor, our higher vantage point was never a point of advantage.

I staked out a position at the end of a long table; an aisle separated us from the next table on our tier. There was only one tier higher than mine, so I was fairly well isolated, and I was confident that I could breathe without emitting any booze fumes.

My favorite course was Contracts I, because of our prestigious and venerable old Professor Jaeger. He was seventy-five years old, but he was possessed of an abundance of energy and a razor-sharp wit. Professor Jaeger was a master storyteller. He liked to remind us that, in 1934, which was his first year as a faculty member at Georgetown Law School, Lyndon Baines Johnson was enrolled at the school. As it turned out, Mr. Johnson, drawn by the allure of politics, dropped out after attending his first semester. I found comfort in that, although I had no illusions that a career in national politics lay ahead of me.

There is no hard and fast rule concerning how many hours students should dedicate to their legal studies. I studied and worked on writing briefs for three hours each weekday morning and spent five hours studying each Saturday and Sunday. I spent four hours in the classroom each weekday afternoon. This amounted to 45 hours each week, about the same number of hours one would spend working a full-time job. I did not feel at all overworked while attending law school.

I became quite skilled at drinking enough to stay brave while avoiding the poor judgment and bad behavior that resulted from drinking too much. It was a fine line that I learned to tread carefully.

I knew that my morning buzz would not be enough to carry me through an entire afternoon. So, I resorted to taping small bottles of vodka just under my calves. These bottles held just under three ounces each. I was fortunate that big, polyester bell-bottoms were in style. These pants effectively concealed any bulges from the reusable, plastic flaskets that would serve me so well.

I'd tape one small bottle to each leg, just above the ankle, to smooth the edges when the effects of the screwdrivers began to wane. After the first class, I would use a restroom stall, remove a bottle from my leg, and reattach it after downing its contents. I would consume the other bottle after my second class. Considering the quantity of vodka I drank, it was amazing that no one ever caught on to what I was doing.

But every day, as I rode the train home from school, I'd experience the dreadful feeling that even if I somehow made it through John Marshall, I'd never be able to practice law. I knew that not too far down the line, I was headed for abject and total failure. I couldn't imagine what my father would think when the truth was finally revealed.

CHAPTER 7

Mom Goes to Rehab (And I Should Have Joined Her)

My mom's drinking finally reached the point where we, her kids, decided she needed to undergo rehab at a hospital. My brother Rick made the arrangements. Mom was admitted to Lutheran General Hospital on Tuesday, November 1, 1977. The hospital was located in the Chicago suburb of Park Ridge, the same town where Hillary Rodham Clinton grew up.

Because of her very heavy drinking and reliance on alcohol, our mother required a medical detox, which meant three to five days of Librium given in doses of 50 milligrams every four hours. A non-medical detox would have been too risky. Many people have died trying to withdraw from alcohol without sedatives or medical supervision.

After she was safely detoxed, my mom received lower doses of benzodiazepines to keep her steady. We made our first visit on her seventh day in rehab. She was still receiving Librium, but it was being tapered to 25 milligrams every six hours. Most patients remained on benzos for seven days to prevent delirium tremens or seizures.

As for me, I was still drinking every weekday morning before law school, and sneaking vodka into the restroom during my breaks between classes. When we left for the hospital at about 6:30 in the evening, I hadn't had a drink for about three-and-a-half hours. By the time we reached the hospital at 7:00, I was coming down hard.

Rick had driven, and along with us were our other six siblings. We met our mom in a visiting area but were soon told that she would be attending an AA meeting, and we were invited to attend an Al-Anon meeting, which provided information for the patients' families.

We entered a room with about fifteen chairs arranged in a circle. The facilitator told us that we were going to take turns reading aloud from some prepared Al-Anon literature. When my turn came, I was shaking so badly that I could barely hold the page I was reading. Somehow, I made it through that meeting, and we spent some time with our mom.

My mother accomplished something amazing after her release from rehab. She maintained her sobriety for four years until she died of colon cancer in June of 1981. I couldn't stay sober for even one day. Just as my mom had required rehab, I surely knew I did as well.

CHAPTER 8

Lovestruck in Law School

In January of my second semester at John Marshall, Abby Gibson, who would never have given me the time of day if I weren't in law school, contacted me through a friend, and we began dating. I was drinking more, and I began acting more brashly at school, demonstrating the haughty self-confidence that vodka encouraged. I welcomed the challenges issued by our professors, and, as far as I could tell, drinking remained my dirty little secret.

But the mornings were getting tougher, and I started drinking before breakfast, and more importantly, before reading my cases and writing my briefs. I knew I was becoming more dependent on alcohol the first morning that I saw my hands trembling until I'd had my morning "eye-opener."

The most glaring indication that I was out of control came when I decided I needed to drink before taking my second-semester finals. Amazingly, I did much better on these exams than I did at the end of my first semester. I credited the vodka, but it was probably due to my getting used to our law school schedule. I knew that I would not be able to continue school drinking every day and that a train wreck lurked around the corner.

I decided to take a semester off to clear my head. This didn't go over well with Abby or, in particular, my father. I couldn't bear the notion of spending another summer with him and Coralee anyway. And as it turned out, if I was not going to continue in school, he was not interested in having me work with him. I knew that he was ashamed of me—he made no attempt to hide it. All I ever had going for me was academic success, and without it, I was nothing, both in his eyes and mine.

I kept Abby from leaving me altogether by guaranteeing that I would only be taking a semester off and would once again be a law student come January. Abby was hard to please. I had to pay for every date, every concert we attended, every restaurant—I paid for everything we did. Then, she told me that I needed to buy a car. After all, she insisted, I was 23 years old, and owning a car was long overdue.

A few months earlier, I had moved into the house that Abby shared with her sister, Bonnie. Abby had been waking early to drive me to a shitty job I'd landed at a factory that made valves and other equipment for public toilets. This job certainly didn't hold the cachet of being a law student, and I lost my ace in the hole as far as attracting women was concerned.

I took out a loan and purchased a 1973 Mercury Montego, white with a black leather top and black leather bucket seats. It was in very good condition, but I was secretly ashamed that my first car was already five years old. At least I had a vehicle, and that was one less thing for Abby to complain about. And her list of complaints was growing.

I knew that she was on the verge of dumping me, and although it stung to realize how little she cared for me, I knew that her reasons for throwing me were sound. I was a mess, and everybody knew it.

The final blow to my wounded psyche came one Saturday morning when I discovered her diary. She had left for the day—she was spending less and less time at her place—and I awoke to learn she was gone. She kept the book in one of her dresser drawers, and I knew I had no business searching for it, but I was desperate. When I found her diary, my heart pounded so fast that I could barely catch my breath. The diary had no lock, and I started thumbing through it, looking for any references to me. My hands were shaking. I expected to find many and was crushed to see that she had only thought to mention me once. Once. She had written page upon page about several different guys. She'd been using this journal for years, and she thought of me one fucking time.

I stared at the only entry that included me. It read, "I've broken so many hearts, and now I'm going to have to hurt Rob. He fell so hard for me. I never meant for that to happen, poor guy."

My stomach was a mess. I felt like throwing up. I didn't know what to think, except that I was finished. "Fuck, she's gonna dump me. What am I going to do without her?"

Abby broke up with me soon after I'd read her diary. She had good reason to be rid of me as my downward spiral continued.

CHAPTER 9

First Rehab

My roommate from college, Mark Tolbert, and I were living in an apartment in Oak Park. I didn't have a job and was collecting a small unemployment check of $160 every other week. So, finances were tight.

Mark was working at a law firm downtown, Wilson, Baker, Whitney, and Gray, but he had received an offer to be a runner at the Board of Trade and decided to take the job. He asked me if I would be interested in replacing him as a clerk at the firm, and I said yes. He spent a week showing me the ins and outs of the job, then he started work at the Board of Trade, and I was on my own. I realized that I would need the help of my old friend, vodka, to do this job.

Fortunately, Mark left for work earlier than I did, so every morning, when I heard his alarm go off, I would reach under my bed for my 1.5-liter bottle of vodka and drink from a mug that I kept in the room. The vodka burned as it went down, but I was used to that, and it became an essential part of my routine.

By the time Mark left for work, I'd have a strong morning buzz. I would shave and shower, but I wouldn't brush my teeth until just before leaving, because I continued to take small slugs of vodka as I prepared for work.

Drinking at work was not fun, but it was necessary. I told myself that I was a "functioning alcoholic," and I did my job as well as I could under the circumstances. But it was only a matter of time before my booze bubble burst, and I would be nailed for drinking on the job. I wondered just how and when that would take place.

Then one day, my house of cards came crashing down. It was 11:00 on a Tuesday morning, February 3, 1981. After I'd finished filing motions and orders at the courthouse, I returned to the office. Andrea, the receptionist, who also happened to be a good friend of Mark, told me that Todd Allen, one of the associates, wanted to see me as soon as I returned. I knew why; I walked to Todd's office and tapped on his open door.

"Rob," he said, "come on in. Close the door, please. We need to talk."

My stomach was in knots. I took a seat.

"Rob, this is very difficult for me, but I have to say it. The partners have asked me to talk to you about your drinking. The word is, you smell of liquor every morning, and it stays with you throughout the day. We know that you are drinking on the job, and we believe you have a serious problem."

I tried to play dumb. "A problem?"

"Rob," he said, "everyone here is very fond of you. You're a smart and personable guy, but we can't ignore this."

"I really don't know what you mean, Todd. Sure, I have to admit that some days I have a beer or two at lunch, but I'm not an alcoholic."

That was pure bullshit, and he wasn't buying it.

"Come on, Rob, level with me. You represent the firm, and this is bad for our image. Fortunately, you're covered under an excellent insurance policy. We'd like you to get help, you know, go to rehab, then come back to work with us as a sober employee. It's the best thing for all of us. What do you say, Rob?"

Cut the crap, I thought. *The jig is up*.

"Yeah, Todd, why lie? I do have a drinking problem, and I think that rehab is the right idea, a chance to start over."

More bullshit. I didn't have any desire to stop drinking. It was the one thing in my life that provided some relief from my infernal anxiety.

"Great. Well, we're going to pay you early. You can pick up your check from Andrea. Then I want you to call the insurance company and get yourself into a hospital as soon as possible."

We shook hands, and I left.

I headed to the receptionist's desk. I wanted out as quickly as possible.

"Andrea, Todd said you had a check for me."

She tried to avoid eye contact.

"Oh yes, here it is," she said.

She handed me a check. I looked at it. Two hundred sixty dollars. I decided that would finance a good bender.

I said goodbye to Andrea and stepped into the elevator. As soon as it reached the ground floor, I went straight to the bank and cashed my check. Then I made a beeline to a dimly lit gin joint to get good and smashed. As long as I had enough money to stay wasted, that was what I was going to do. I spent the next few days drinking at the apartment until late afternoon, when I would leave and visit the many taverns in the neighboring suburb of Forest Park.

By Thursday morning, I had burned through almost $200, and I was in a fix. The rent was due that day, February 5. I went into Mark's room, and on his dresser were $150 and a note asking me to combine his share with mine to pay the owner our February rent. Of course, my half of the rent was just about gone. I would be busted by Mark, and we would have a very angry landlady to deal with. I needed a plan. Then, it came to me. I would take Mark's $150, combine it with my remaining cash, and treat myself to a sumptuously expensive restaurant meal. Then I would buy a fifth of Stolichnaya, the good stuff, ingest one hundred over-the-counter sleeping pills, and go to sleep permanently.

I enjoyed my lavish dinner, and the bill came to $180, including drinks and a generous tip. I returned home late that night and carried out the next stage of my plan. I ingested every pill and washed it down with half a fifth of Stoli.

Despite my plan, I awoke at dawn on Saturday. My strategy had failed—I was still alive. I managed to avoid Mark until Sunday evening, when he told me that he knew that I'd been busted at work. I made up some cockamamie story that I had somehow lost the rent money. That was a whopper, and Mark wasn't having any of it.

Mark called my family, and the next morning, Monday, February 9, my brother Rick arrived to take me to the University of Illinois Hospital for a 28-day detox and rehab. I showered and dressed, and I was off to begin my stay at what would be the first of several alcohol rehabs.

CHAPTER 10

Water Street Market

It was the midsummer of 1981, and I was living rent-free with my brother Ray and our good friend, Steve. I needed to find a job and earn enough money to quit sponging off of them and get a place of my own. I checked the classifieds daily, searching for factory or warehouse work. I didn't have many other skills to offer an employer.

The classifieds weren't brimming with work for which I was qualified. There were a bunch of telephone sales positions, but I wanted nothing to do with cold-calling people at dinner time and having the phone slammed down in my ear.

Each Monday, I'd wake up early, about 6:00 a.m., shower, and head out the door, with the Sunday Tribune classifieds tucked under my arm. I didn't know where I was headed, but I wanted Ray and Steve to know that I was at least trying to find a job.

For a week, I rode the bus to various industrial parks scattered throughout the city. I had to budget the little money I had, and I would make do with an Egg-McMuffin and a glass of water for breakfast. Later in the afternoon, before heading back to Ray and Steve's, I would once again hit the McDonald's for a plain burger and another water.

Finally, on the first Sunday of August, I spotted a help-wanted ad for a produce clerk at a place called Alberti's, a fruit and vegetable wholesaler at the Water Street Market, a Chicago landmark known for its frenetic pace and the pre-dawn mayhem that occurred Monday through Friday. This was my first opportunity to land a stable, well-paying job.

The ad specified that interested applicants should apply between 10:00 and noon on Monday, August 3. That's probably when the craziness of the early morning began to wind down. There would likely be a swarm of applicants. I'd need to arrive well before 10:00 and impress my potential employer with my punctuality.

That Sunday afternoon, while Ray and Steve were gone, I sneaked out to the liquor store and purchased a pint of vodka. I would need my trusty bottle of bravery before encountering the madness that was Water Market Street.

I got back to the apartment and hid the bottle under the couch that also served as my bed. I was dying for a small taste, just enough to take the edge off, but I knew I would need every bit of that pint to get through the following day.

I woke at seven. Steve was already dressed and enjoying his breakfast. He always left for work at 7:30. Ray was a bartender at a trendy Italian restaurant on Superior, just east of Michigan Avenue. He'd leave the apartment at 9:30 to show up in time to prep and open the bar by 11:00. So, while Steve ate breakfast, I shaved and showered so I could stay out of Ray's way.

Ray woke at about 8:30, drank his morning cup of coffee, and headed to the bathroom. This was my chance. I reached deep under the couch and retrieved my pint of vodka. I quickly tucked it under a cushion and waited until I heard Ray start the shower. I got a glass of ice water, returned to the couch, and grabbed the bottle. I was really on edge, keeping an ear open in case Ray ended his shower early. I unscrewed the bottle's red plastic cap, took a big, long pull, and swallowed. The low-end vodka burned my throat. I used the ice water to chase it down and finished the pint within a few minutes.

When Ray left the shower for his bedroom, I darted into the bathroom, brushed my teeth, and, for good measure, swallowed a glob of toothpaste. Ray was still in his room when I reached the front door and shouted goodbye. I bolted down the front steps with the empty bottle stuffed in a paper bag and rushed out of the lobby.

I walked two blocks to the bus stop at Halsted and Armitage and dumped the bag in a trash can. One of the best things about Chicago was the frequency with which its buses and trains ran. During morning rush hour, the southbound Halsted bus that I would need to take ran roughly every eight minutes.

Shortly after I arrived at the stop, a bus approached. I boarded it and dropped ninety cents into the farebox. I looked at my watch. It was 9:06. Perfect. I would make it to Water Market Street by 9:30.

It was a straight shot south, just past the Lake Street elevated train tracks, known to Chicagoans as the "L." In less than twenty minutes, I exited the bus at the corner of Halsted and West 14th Place. There had been no actual Water Market Street since the 1920s, when the old one was demolished to make way for the splendor of the high-rises of Wacker Drive and Michigan Avenue. The new "Water Market Street" was about two blocks west of Halsted, between 14th Place and West 15th Street. It ran about four city blocks between Morgan Street and Racine Avenue. There were produce markets as far as the eye could see; the place was huge and extremely busy.

It was not even 9:30. I could take my time walking to Alberti's

Wholesale Fruits and Vegetables. I would keep to my plan and wait until 9:45 to enter the office.

The harsh odors of the street assaulted me. The redolence of onions, garlic, and all things noxious permeated the air and bombarded my senses. Probably the most overpowering aroma came from the ammonia that the wholesalers used to wash rotting fruits and vegetables off the pavement and into the sewers.

I was struck by how noisy and chaotic everything was. But this place had been in operation for decades, and I assumed that the street possessed its own set of rules and regulations.

Trucks were coming and going constantly. I thought they were moving too fast through such a busy and crowded location. On every dock, forklifts buzzed to and fro, loading and unloading the trucks. Everyone hollered at the top of their lungs. And they cursed—every other word was an obscenity.

I followed the lot numbers until I arrived at my destination. This place was insane. But I was the one who was jacked up on vodka for a job interview, so who was I to weigh in on sanity? I leaned against a wall as I marveled at the bedlam and listened to the non-stop string of exclamations and expletives.

By 9:45, I was struck by the degree to which the entire street had grown quiet, almost serene. It was time to apply for the job.

I asked a big, round Italian guy where the office was. He just spat and pointed past the forklifts. I walked a short distance until I came to an office. A sign read: "PLEASE KNOCK", so I did.

A handsome young guy with wavy black hair, wearing a white short-sleeved Oxford shirt and a loosened black tie, motioned me inside. I opened the door and entered his office. I was glad I'd arrived early. I was the only applicant there.

"You here about the clerking gig?" he asked.

I tried to sound confident. "Yes, I am," I said.

"Okay, take this clipboard and have a seat over there." He gestured toward an old, red chair. The fabric upholstery was threadbare and dirty. I grabbed the clipboard and took a seat. I removed a pen from my shirt pocket.

"Good, you have your own pen. I like that. My dad always says, 'Never hire anyone who doesn't bring his own pen.' Good advice. My name's Mike, Mike Alberti. My old man owns the place, but he's not around much. Before him, my grandfather ran things, and his father before him."

I rose to shake his hand and wasn't surprised by his firm grip.

"I'm Robert. It's nice to meet you."

"Likewise." He smiled. His teeth were sparkling white.

I had brought a list of previous employers and references so I could get through the application quickly. It took me about ten minutes to complete. I handed him the application form.

"That was quick. You sure you got everything?"

"Pretty sure. Yeah."

I didn't list the law firm where I had worked. That would just have invited questions that I didn't have answers for.

"Okay, so you've done a lot of shipping and receiving. Good. That's what we're looking for. I gotta ask you this. How's your sense of humor?"

"My sense of humor? Hmm . . . pretty good, I think. I like a good joke, and I try not to take myself too seriously. Well, that is, I am serious when I have a job to do, so—"

He interrupted me. "Good, cuz you're gonna need a sense of humor to work here. And a thick skin. These drivers are always in a rush, and they're always cussing. They'll yell at you and swear like fucking sailors, but the trick is to not take them seriously. That's just their, um, modus operandi, their M.O."

"Spoken like a true lawyer," I said.

"Hey, you want a job or what? Spoken like a fuckin' lawyer. Shit. Fucking shysters."

"Sorry. I didn't mean anything."

He laughed. "Hey, it's all right. I'm just yankin' your chain. Don't worry. I was just giving you a dose of the daily medicine you're gonna get around here."

He must have grown up in that crazy environment, and he was right at home amid the pandemonium.

"Well, Robert, the job's yours if you want it. Starting pay is twelve bucks an hour. After a month, we put you on our insurance. We start at 4:00 a.m., sharp. I'll see you tomorrow morning."

We shook hands, and I left. I was jubilant. But in the back of my mind, a voice of sad reason told me that this was not something I could do sober. I forced that thought out of my head, walked to Halsted Street, and looked for the nearest tavern to celebrate my good fortune. I looked forward to sharing the good news with Ray and Steve. They were happy to learn that I'd landed a well-paying job and would hopefully stop leeching off of them. I went to bed early; I'd have to be up before 3:00.

The next morning, I rose early, brushed my teeth, and showered. To save time, I had shaved the night before. I left the house at 3:20 and walked to Halsted Street to catch the bus. I was sober, shaking, and scared to death. I knew that I did not have the toughness to handle the job. But I could not have Mike calling the apartment to find out why I hadn't reported for my first day at work. I found a payphone and called Alberti's. When Mike answered the phone, I almost hung up. But I knew what I had to do, so I spoke quickly.

"Hey Mike," I said. "I hate to do this to you, but I'm not coming in."

"What?" he asked. "You told me you wanted this fucking job.

What the fuck is wrong with you?"

"I got a call from another place. I start work there today."

"You're a fucking piece of work, you know that? You're really screwing me. You know what—fuck you." He slammed down the phone.

I was shaken up, but I had done what I had to. If Ray and Steve got a call from him asking where I was, my entire story would have collapsed. I walked back to their building. There was an old couch on the back porch where I curled up and went to sleep. I slept off and on until 9:30, when I was sure that both Ray and Steve had left for work.

I knew I had to find a job, any job. I went into the apartment, opened the newspaper to the classified section, and noticed an ad for a shipping and receiving clerk at a small store on South Halsted. The place, called Evergreen Tools, was a mail-order company that sold woodworking accessories.

I boarded another Halted Street bus, this time exiting at Madison Street. The place was located smack dab in the middle of Chicago's infamous Skid Row.

Evergreen was a modest storefront business with a not-so-roomy work area. The only person in the place when I arrived was the owner, whose name was Sherwin Fischer. He was a peculiar little man who needed someone to fill the warehouse position immediately. I quickly filled out a short application.

He looked it over and said, "I only need one employee to help me run this business. I'll write up the orders, and you'll serve as the order puller, as well as the shipping and receiving clerk. Do you think you can manage that?"

"Sure," I said. "I can definitely handle those tasks."

"If you can start tomorrow morning, the job is yours. The pay is $5.00 an hour. The hours are 8:00 a.m. to 4:30 p.m., with a half-hour lunch."

"Sure, I can start tomorrow. No problem."

"Okay then. Consider yourself hired. Be here on time."

"Thank you," I said. "You won't regret this."

I couldn't believe my luck. I would be working pretty much on my own for this eccentric gentleman who, I soon discovered, called the place home. By that, I meant that he lived in the back room with just a twin bed, a dresser, a hot plate, a toilet, and a sink.

I was soon back on a northbound bus and headed to Ray and Steve's apartment. I would tell them that the Water Market position didn't pan out. I started at Evergreen the next morning.

Right off the bat, I learned that Sherwin was the epitome of a micromanager, who was constantly scrutinizing my work. And because he didn't have a bathtub or shower, he smelled pretty ripe. I did my work, and he was satisfied with my performance. But by the end of my first week, I knew that I could not continue working for this creepy, smelly screwball.

As it turned out, the following Sunday, I found an ad for a receiving clerk at a screw and bolt company in Chicago's Lakeview neighborhood, not far from Ray and Steve's place in Lincoln Park. They were accepting walk-in applicants on Monday morning, August 10. I rose early that Monday, and at 8:00, I called Evergreen to tell Sherwin that I was sick and would not be coming in. He did not take the news well and promptly fired me.

"You can come in Friday afternoon to get your check," he said.

I was good with that. I showered and shaved, and was out the door. By 8:45, I was on a Halsted bus northbound to Diversey. I boarded a second bus for the mile-long trip to Southport, which was two blocks from my destination, Select Screw and Bolt Company. I entered the lobby at 9:15.

There were two men hurriedly filling out their applications. I stepped up to the window, and a young woman asked if I wanted an application. I said yes, and she handed me the paperwork on a clipboard with a pen attached. I rushed through the application and finished ahead of the two men who'd arrived before me. I handed it to the woman behind the window.

"Do you have time to stay for an interview with our personnel manager?" she asked me.

"Yes," I said nervously, "I can stay for an interview."

Within minutes, a stern-looking woman opened the door to the lobby. She called my name.

"That's me. I'm Robert."

"Hello, Robert, my name is Vera. Please follow me."

We walked inside, and she motioned me into her sparsely decorated office. I must have made a good impression because she offered me the job after reviewing my application.

"I believe you have the necessary skills for the receiving position," she said. "The starting pay is $6.00 an hour. After a ninety-day probation period, you'll receive a fifty-cent raise and full health insurance benefits. How does that sound?"

"It sounds very generous," I said.

"Can you start tomorrow at 8:00?"

"Yes, ma'am," I said. "I can start first thing in the morning."

"Very good, then. We'll see you tomorrow. I'll walk you out. Oh, and don't say anything to the other applicants. I'll take care of that."

As she escorted me to the door, I couldn't believe I'd landed my third job in eight days.

I began the next day, and immediately after work on Friday, August 14, I purchased a half-pint of vodka at a corner store and a large Coke at a nearby McDonald's. I ducked into the restroom, poured out some Coke, and topped off the rest with a good measure of vodka. I drank the vodka and Coke as I rode the bus to pick up my paycheck from Sherwin. I knew that the store would be closed, but I hoped that I could still get the check, seeing as he lived there.

By the time I reached the store, I had a pretty good buzz. Sherwin noticed me waiting at the door and approached with my paycheck in hand. I took it from him and thanked him. The check was for $108. He didn't say a word, which was fine with me.

As I headed to the bus stop, a scraggly old bum asked me for some spare change, and I did him one better. He was standing right outside of a dimly lit liquor store. I went inside and purchased a 750-milliliter bottle of Thunderbird, the classic "bum wine." It cost me sixty cents.

As I exited the store and showed the gentleman the bottle I'd bought for him, he gave me a toothless smile and said, "What's the word? Thunderbird. How's it sold? Good and cold."

I laughed, and he invited me to share the bottle with him. Not wanting to contract hepatitis or some other type of cootie, I opened the bottle and took the first slug. Then I handed it to my new friend and said, "It's all yours, my good man. Enjoy."

"You're an A-1, bona fide gentleman," he said. I shook his hand and boarded a bus. I had done my good deed for the day.

CHAPTER 11

The Maybrook Hotel

After working two weeks at my new job at Select Screw and Bolt, I received my first four-day paycheck, $166.00 after taxes. I moved out of Ray and Steve's apartment and got a room at the Maybrook Hotel, a dumpy SRO on Diversey Parkway, just a short walk to work. The rent was $40 a week; I was certainly not living in the lap of luxury. My room had a sink with separate hot and cold faucets, and everyone shared the bathroom down the hall. Usually, if I had to take a leak, I just pissed in my sink.

I didn't want any of my warehouse buddies to know that I lived in that decrepit hotel just down the alley from Select. So, each day after work, I would head down Racine to the Lincoln Park area with all its hip bars and eateries. When I was sufficiently buzzed, I would walk back to the Maybrook, piss in the sink, and go to sleep.

Leaving the hotel for work in the morning was tricky. The front entrance was in plain sight of everybody who used Diversey to drive to work. At first, I would leave early and walk the neighborhood, but there were a handful of employees who showed up early each day, and I didn't want any of them to spot me sneaking out of my seedy digs.

I decided it would be a good idea to drink a few screwdrivers each morning. Not too many, just enough to boost my confidence.

Sufficiently buzzed, I would crawl out my third-floor window, which faced the alley. Then I'd scurry down the fire escape, hang from the landing grate that was ten feet high, and drop to the ground.

This system worked fairly well, but before long, I was getting the shakes as lunchtime approached. I had a remedy for this, though. There was a corner store owned by two Palestinian brothers, and at lunch, I would rush to the store and make my daily purchase of a quart of beer and a half-pint of peppermint schnapps.

The brothers, who I was pretty sure never touched alcohol, were very courteous when I arrived each afternoon to purchase my liquid lunch. After paying my bill, I'd hustle to the alley where, as luck would have it, there stood the dilapidated remains of an old garage. There was not a lick of paint left, and the wood had assumed a grayish color. I would sneak in, slam down the Schnapps in three gulps, then enjoy my quart of beer, which I would consume in about 15 minutes. I would then return to work, fortified for the next few hours.

My routine worked smoothly for a few months, until one very cold January morning in 1982. It was a Thursday. I was enjoying my morning cocktails when I crossed the line between buzzed and sloppy drunk. I should have skipped work and called in sick from the payphone in the hotel lobby. But I was so drunk that I reasoned I could go to work and do my job without anyone noticing how shit-faced I was.

I walked to the window, opened it, and crawled through. I kind of just dropped to the third-floor landing and laughed. I was in a very good, very drunken mood. I got up and closed the window. Then, I proceeded to hug the rail as I took the steps to the second-floor landing. Next, I grabbed the grate and hung by both arms above the pavement.

Splat! I landed safely on my ass in that grimy little alley. I was beaming with good cheer as I staggered to work. I punched in just after 8:00 and walked to a pallet that held nine full kegs of screws. I was supposed to check each keg to make sure the screws were the correct type and in good condition. Next, I was supposed to drive a forklift and bring the pallet to a large scale to make sure we'd received the right amount of screws.

But before I made it to an available forklift, I was stopped by Curtis, our receiving foreman. Curtis was a big, strong Black man who sported a smoothly shaved head. He conducted himself with an air of quiet confidence and authority.

"Rob, my man," Curtis said. "Have you been drinking this morning?"

I confessed immediately.

"Ya know, Rob, why don't you sit at my desk while I go talk to Matt?"

Matt Lewis was the plant manager. I knew I was screwed. But I did as I was told, and Curtis went to find him.

As I was about to nod off, I could see Curtis and Matt approaching. They were accompanied by Brent and Natalie Cabot, the brother and sister owners, as well as Vera, the no-nonsense personnel manager.

Brent spoke first.

"Robert, it looks like you're pretty intoxicated. Why don't you come with us?"

The six of us left the receiving area and walked through the large packaging area to a set of stairs that led to the purchasing department. We walked to the purchasing director's office. Brent knocked, and Dan Foster, the purchasing director, opened the door.

"Let's go to the conference room," Dan said.

We reached a large room with a long maple table.

"Let's everyone have a seat," Natalie said.

So, we all sat.

Vera turned to me. "Robert, it's obvious to everyone here that you are very inebriated. Do you admit that you've been drinking?"

I knew I was fucked. What could I say?

"Robert, everyone at Select likes you and knows that you're a good worker, but this is a serious breach of company policy," Vera continued.

Natalie weighed in. "Robert, we think it would be a good idea for you to take today and tomorrow off and return to work sober on Monday morning."

"You mean I'm not fired?" I asked.

"No," Brent said, "but this is a one-time warning. Next time, we will have to let you go."

A phone rang, and Dan answered it. "The cab's here," he said.

"Fine," Matt said. "Let's walk Robert to his taxi."

So, Curtis, Matt, and I headed down the stairs and walked to the receiving ramp, where a Yellow Taxi was waiting.

Matt gave the driver ten bucks. "Take this gentleman home, and please don't make any stops," he said. "You can keep the change."

The driver took the bill. I got in, fastened my seat belt, and gave him Ray and Steve's address.

"See you Monday. Bright-eyed and bushy-tailed," Curtis said. I liked Curtis and knew he was just doing his job.

When we got to the apartment, about three miles away, I got out of the cab. *God*, I prayed, *please don't let Ray see me like this.*

To my relief, no one was around. The cab drove off, and I headed to Halsted and walked north for a while until I reached some dive bar, went in, and ordered a bottle of Michelob and a shot of Jack Daniel's. I left the bar in search of a liquor store. I made my way east on Diversey until I found a Walgreens where I purchased two fifths of vodka, a bottle of grapefruit juice, and a twelve-pack of Old Style. I boarded a westbound bus to the Maybrook and reached the hotel just before noon. I decided to finish the beer and vodka by Saturday, then sober up on Sunday.

Somehow, I made it from Saturday afternoon to Monday morning without a drink. I was very shaky, but I was sober. I nervously took the fire escape down to the alley and walked to Select. I never drank on a workday morning for the rest of my time there.

A few months went by, and I was weighing some kegs when Dan Foster showed up.

"How's it going, Robert? Vendors not ripping us off?"

"Oh, hi, Dan. You can call me Rob," I said.

"Okay, Rob. Did you happen to see the graffiti in the men's room under the purchasing department?"

"Be alert," I said, "this company needs more lerts."

Dan laughed. "Yeah, that's the one," he said. "Pretty funny."

I smiled. "Yeah. I wrote that. I saw it in the library restroom when I was going to the U. of I. I thought it was funny too."

"You went to the U. of I.? In Champaign?"

"Yeah."

"Then why in the fuck are you working in a warehouse counting fucking screws and bolts?"

"It's kind of a long story," I said.

"I'll bet it is. Anyway, Brent Cabot saw what you wrote, and, man, was he ever pissed. Nice work, Rob. You really got under his skin."

I smiled again. "Thanks."

"Don't worry. I won't tell him it was you. I want him to go apeshit trying to figure out who the Graffiti Bandit is. You know he'd fire your ass if he found out."

"Yeah, I kinda figured," I said.

"So, you went to the University of Illinois, and now you work in a fucking warehouse."

"Pretty much my story. Yep."

"Well, I may have a remedy for that. How would you like to come up to purchasing? Be a buyer. Probably not much more pay, but it's cleaner and easier on the back."

"You could do that?"

"Sure. I'll talk to Natalie. She likes you."

"I don't know how Curtis is gonna feel about me jumping ahead of him."

"You don't have to worry about Curtis. But you do have to worry about me. I'm a fifth-degree black belt in karate, and if I ever smell booze on your breath, I'll break both your legs."

He turned and walked away.

Just days after our conversation, Dan asked if I was ready to move to purchasing. I certainly was.

Soon after I went to purchasing, Rosemary Jansen was bumped up to buyer as well. She was cute, not beautiful, but cute. Rosemary was a smoker, about a pack a day, but she had the whitest teeth. And this was before the whole tooth-whitening thing came into vogue.

Sadly, Dan and his wife decided to move to Hawaii, and Dennis, a friend of the Cabots, was hired as our new purchasing director. Eileen, who had been in purchasing the longest, really should have received the promotion, but she was kind of pushy and not at all attractive, and the Cabots put a premium on good looks. So, she got screwed.

We had a purchasing department of four buyers, Rosemary, Eileen, Sharon, and me, along with our fearless leader, Dennis. It came as no surprise that Dennis was a regular drinking buddy of Natalie and Brent.

Every morning, Dennis would arrive a little late to work. His eyes were always glassy and bloodshot, and his breath reeked of the stale booze that he had probably consumed just a few hours earlier.

Dennis had no idea how to buy nuts and bolts or keep up with stock status and inventory reports. But Eileen was happy to jump in, and she became our *de facto* director after all. Dennis would pretty much just stay in his office until lunch, which, I believed, was liquid.

I missed Dan. He was a good boss and fun to be around. But with Dennis at the helm, I reasoned I could hang out after work with my old buddies from the warehouse and drink some beers at quitting time. On Fridays, we would all head to Riley's, which was a bar located directly across the street from my hotel. We would drink, listen to the jukebox, and play shuffleboard bowling for beers.

Curtis would always leave after just a few drinks. He had a girlfriend and preferred spending Friday nights with her. The rest of us would leave at about 6:30 or 7:00. Mike Castro and I would usually leave together and head to the new-wave bars like NEO and Club 950. The rest of the guys were into heavy metal and hated new-wave music.

Every Saturday morning, I'd wake up hungover and figure out how much money I'd blown the night before. It was usually about sixty dollars—far more than I could afford to spend in one night. I'd promise myself to spend my money more judiciously the following Friday. But every Saturday morning, I was sixty dollars poorer.

My routine was to drink heavily Friday night, continue drinking vodka alone in my room early Saturday morning, then head to a dive bar next to the Diversey L station. I always stopped my drinking at 2:00 each Sunday afternoon, but the hangover and shakes would be there to greet me every Monday morning.

I was growing tired of going to work each morning with the shakes, but as soon as I got off work, I'd make a beeline to the loading dock to drink beer with the boys. I was trapped in an alcoholic quagmire, and I didn't know how to break free.

CHAPTER 12

Adventures on Broadway

Despite my wasteful Friday night spending and drinking sprees, I was able to put away about forty or fifty bucks a week working at Select. I received a raise when I was promoted to purchasing; it was not a great deal. I was only making $7.00 an hour, but I had no expenses except the $40.00 weekly rent at the Maybrook.

By March of 1982, I had managed to save just over a thousand dollars. I found a studio apartment on Roscoe Street in Chicago's East Lakeview neighborhood. The rent was $225.00 a month, and I paid one month's security deposit. This meant that for the modest sum of $450.00, I was able to say goodbye to the Maybrook.

The building on Roscoe was constructed in the early 1960s and was known as a "4 + 1," which meant that the first floor consisted of a slab of concrete that was used for parking spaces. Above the garage were four floors of apartments. So, it was actually a five-story building with parking, a lobby, and laundry facilities on the first floor.

I bought a simple metal-framed trundle bed, a particleboard shelf unit, and a small black and white TV from a nearby Goodwill. I purchased a small kitchen table and four blue fabric director chairs from Sears. My place was humble, but it was home.

Back in 1982, the neighborhood was quite seedy. It was

inhabited by an army of hookers, homeless people, and a very large number of mentally ill patients who had been deinstitutionalized—that is, set free—in the late 1960s and early 1970s. These people, who wandered the streets without any direction, made living in East Lakeview an adventure I could have done without.

One warm spring morning, a Monday, I was sitting quietly on the Southbound Broadway bus, on the way to work. I was jonesing pretty bad after a weekend of non-stop boozing. I stared at the floor, trying to avoid eye contact with any other riders, when a mentally ill man took a seat next to me. He was wearing a heavy winter coat and a pair of cloth gloves that were missing the fingers.

"I like your shoes. You have nice shoes," he said.

Oh shit, I thought.

"Thank you. I'm glad you like them."

"Do you think I could try them on? Please? I'd really like to try them on."

"Sorry, my stop is coming up."

To my extreme horror, the man knelt on the floor and began to untie one of my shoes. Everybody was watching. Fuck, I was under a most unwelcome spotlight. I pulled my foot away from him, but he was persistent. He continued yanking on the laces.

"You can't have my fucking shoes. Now, please move. I have to get off this bus!"

I was surprised when he backed off. He stood up and said, "I'm sorry. I hope you're not mad at me. I just like your shoes."

I felt like a heartless piece of shit. "I'm sorry," I said, "I shouldn't have yelled at you."

He walked away crestfallen, poor guy. The bus stopped, and I skulked away.

***

On a crisp Sunday morning in early April, I awoke at 4:00 and decided to have a few drinks. I opted for screwdrivers and quickly downed two very strong cocktails. By far, the best thing about my tiny apartment on Roscoe Street was its proximity to the lakeshore. I decided to take a short walk, less than a quarter-mile, and watch the sun rise over Lake Michigan. I was feeling pretty mellow when the glass slipped out of my hand, hit the counter, shattered, and landed on my right foot. There was a lot of blood, but the booze lessened the sting. I examined the wound. It was pretty large, about two inches long, and quite deep. There were also small shards of glass embedded in the gash. I knew I needed stitches, so I wrapped my foot in a dish towel, grabbed my keys and wallet, and took the elevator from my fifth-floor apartment to the lobby.

I reached the lobby and walked toward Broadway to catch a cab to the hospital. I made it to the corner of Roscoe and Broadway and sat on the curb. The sun had not yet begun to rise, and the street was deserted.

I caught sight of two women—hookers, no doubt—and they could see that I was hurt.

"What's wrong, baby?" one of them asked.

They were both very attractive, and they were wearing tight, short skirts and faux fur coats. And makeup, lots of makeup.

"Damn, honey, what happened?" one of them asked.

I looked up and grimaced. "I dropped a glass on my foot. The cut's pretty deep."

"Let me see how bad it is," she said.

She sat on the curb beside me and unwrapped the towel. "Damn," she said. "You need stitches, baby. Do you have a car?"

"No. No, I don't."

"And there's not one damn cab on the street. I'll use a pay phone to call one," said the other girl.

"Thanks," I said.

Just then, a small Datsun hatchback pulled up. Inside was a

very pretty, very preppy young woman. The hookers waved her down. I wondered what she was doing out alone in this neighborhood so early in the morning.

"Say, honey. Our friend needs to go to the hospital for stitches. He's cut real bad."

The girl looked nervous, but for some inexplicable reason, she agreed to give me a ride.

"I can drive you to Saint Joseph's," she said. "It's the nearest hospital."

I was buzzed, but not drunk. The hookers hadn't made me nervous, but this elegant young woman was a different story. She was just the type of girl I was attracted to. Young, pretty, conservative dresser. Conservative but stylish.

She leaned over and opened the passenger door. I got in.

"Hi, I'm Margaret. How are you feeling?"

I turned my head to the window. I didn't want to blow booze breath on her.

"Hi, Margaret. My name's Rob. I'm good. Thanks so much for doing this."

"Oh, no problem. You need to get to a hospital. I must say, you have some colorful friends."

I blushed. "They were really nice," I said.

We drove off, and I waved to my new friends.

"Thanks, ladies, for everything."

"Not a problem, honey. You take care of yourself," they shouted.

The ride wasn't long, but I struggled to make conversation. As we pulled up to the emergency room, I said, "Thank you so much, Margaret. I'll be fine from here."

"You're very welcome, Rob. I guess I'll be leaving."

She drove off. I never saw Margaret or the hookers again.

CHAPTER 13

My First Shrink

By the spring of 1983, I was growing weary of my daily pattern of drinking and jonesing, drinking and jonesing. I wanted to quit for good, but I kept putting it off. I decided that drinking was not working for me when, in a drunken stupor after a Friday evening of heavy drinking, I boarded an "L" train home. The problem was, I had mistakenly taken a train headed downtown. As the train stopped at State and Lake, I discovered that I had vomited all over myself, as well as my seat and the floor. I could barely see. I touched my face to make sure I was wearing my glasses. I wasn't. I searched through the mess and could not find them. My best guess was that someone whom I had offended with my drunken display had taken them off my face and exited the train with my spectacles. Good punishment for bad behavior.

I stumbled onto a northbound train, which took me to the Diversey stop, and I managed the mile-and-a-half walk from the L station to my apartment on Roscoe Street.

I did not have a spare pair of glasses, and when I arrived at work on Monday morning, I explained to Daniel Mendoza, one of my friends from the warehouse, that I had lost them Friday evening. He told me he had an old pair that were no longer strong enough, and he offered to let me have them.

After work, he drove me to his apartment to get his old glasses. Daniel lived with his wife, Neva, and five-year-old son, Samuel. Neva was a strikingly beautiful young Hispanic woman. On meeting her, I could not for the life of me understand why Daniel would spend all his time getting drunk with his co-workers when he could be spending time with his wife and son. I reasoned that drinking was more important to him than his family. He offered me a ride home, but I could see that Neva didn't want him to leave. So, I said thanks, but I could get home on my own. I stopped on the way to buy my regular six-pack of 16-ounce Old Styles.

The glasses worked well. I planned to keep the slightly dated spectacles until I could afford a new pair. When I showed up to work Tuesday morning with my "new" glasses, Daniel loudly announced my arrival. "Hey, everyone, it's Conan the Librarian."

Everybody laughed. I was embarrassed but tried to be a good sport. After all, he had given me a perfectly good pair of glasses. Besides, what he said was pretty funny, and I didn't have a good comeback.

That entire day, I felt miserable. I wanted a drink so bad, and at lunch, I almost slipped out to buy the quart of beer and half-pint of schnapps I used to drink when I was still working in the warehouse. I managed to tough it out, and later that day, I checked the Yellow Pages for a list of nearby psychiatrists. I found a doctor at Illinois Masonic Hospital, which was within walking distance of work. I made an appointment for lunchtime the following day, March 9. I told Dennis that I had a doctor's appointment. That was all he or anyone else needed to know. The only person who knew the truth was Rosemary. I trusted her, and I knew that she would support me. Although I tried to resist the temptation to drink after work that day, I bought a six-pack of Old Styles and drank them all.

I awoke Wednesday morning, shaky as usual, and immediately

remembered my psychiatrist appointment. I was too nervous to eat breakfast. I shaved and showered, and carefully chose what I hoped were the appropriate clothes for meeting a shrink. I laughed to myself at how dumb an idea it was to think that certain clothes were more or less appropriate to wear for a session with a psychiatrist.

I walked a block and boarded a southbound Broadway Avenue bus. As usual, I checked my seat carefully to make sure that it was clean, or more precisely, that it had not been pissed on. I arrived at work at my usual time and headed upstairs to the purchasing department. Eileen welcomed me.

"Hey, handsome. All set for your doctor's appointment?"

I liked Eileen and felt kind of sorry for her. The Cabots thought she was overbearing and unprofessional. They hadn't given her the director's job when Dan left, because they didn't want her to be the "face" of Select Screw and Bolt.

Eileen was very capable, but she had some rough edges. And, while she wasn't fat, she had a sturdy figure. Her legs were strong, and some of the warehouse guys remarked favorably about them. While some people thought she was butch, I knew she wasn't. I could tell that she was attracted to men. She would have been better off if she had let her short hair grow and focused on improving her complexion.

"So," she said, "big appointment today. What's up with that?"

"Terminal cancer," I said. I didn't want to discuss it.

"Hmm . . . touchy, touchy. What—are you seeing a shrink or something?"

"Yes, Eileen, I am going to see a shrink because working with you is driving me crazy."

She got the joke.

Rosemary arrived and didn't mention my appointment. Rosemary was great, and she possessed a perkiness and charm that made her more attractive. Almost every guy in the warehouse had a thing for Rosemary. I was developing a crush on her myself. She was dating a Chicago cop, but it didn't seem to me that she was madly in love with him or anything.

As usual, the last to arrive was Dennis. It was not merely his breath that reeked of stale booze, but his pores seemed to ooze alcohol as well. Dennis preferred to arrive without fanfare. He would deliver a subdued hello, grab a cup of coffee, and slink into his office to try and regroup from a night of heavy drinking. *Man,* I thought, *if I were Dennis, the last thing I'd want would be a cup of coffee.*

After he had collected himself, Dennis would call Eileen into his office and ask what needed to be done. She relished this because Dennis would delegate all the work to her, and she would convey his plans to us. Rosemary and I knew what to do, so we blew her off and did our jobs our way.

My appointment was at 11:30. At 11:00, I announced that I was leaving. Rosemary gave me a look of support. "Good luck, Bucko." I liked it when she called me Bucko.

I headed downstairs and through the warehouse. I was very nervous about meeting the doctor. My memory took me back to April of 1981, when my mom was still alive, and I started seeing a therapist. She was a psychologist, and she was beautiful. One afternoon, I showed up drunk to an appointment. She told me that she could not see me if I was drinking. I left and never returned.

And there I was, walking to my appointment with a goddamn psychiatrist, Dr. Benjamin Drexel. After a ten-minute walk, I reached the grounds of the hospital and walked until I spotted a sign for the outpatient behavioral health department. I found Dr. Drexel's name in the directory; his office was on the second floor. I considered turning around and walking out, and probably would have skipped the appointment if I hadn't told Rosemary about it. She liked me and was concerned about my drinking and unhealthy lifestyle. Rosemary didn't come straight out and say it, but it was pretty clear she thought I had a drinking problem. So, there was no turning back. Not if I wanted to save face with Rosemary. And, as I assessed my life, I knew it was going nowhere if I didn't stop drinking.

I was flooded with emotions as I recalled something my mom had said to me when I was ten. She was pretty drunk, and we were walking to Walgreens, where she would stock up on booze. I was with her to help carry the packages of liquor and beer. I hated going to Walgreens with my mom when she was on a bender.

I said something—I don't remember exactly what—but it was probably something like I wish we didn't have to go. Couldn't she stop drinking? Wouldn't she? Please?

She did not like that kind of talk, but her reaction floored me. "You know what," she said, "you need to see a psychiatrist. You really do. Something's not right with your head."

Her remark stung like a slap in the face, but I shook it off and didn't say a word the rest of the way.

Eventually, we arrived at Walgreens. She made a beeline for the liquor department, and I headed to the comic-book vending machines. The Walgreens had two machines that stood side by side. One had all the superhero comic books, *Superman*, *Batman*, *Green Lantern*, and such. I didn't care for those comics. The other machine had my favorites—*Archie, Richie Rich, Little Lotta, Little Dot, Casper*, and *Sad Sack,* to name a few. I liked the funny comic books. At least I thought they were funny when I was ten.

In 1965, comic books cost twelve cents. The machines had coin mechanisms similar to those of washing machines in a laundromat. Each featured comic book had its own mechanism. You'd select your comic, insert a dime and two pennies into a tray, slide it into the machine, pull it back out, and the comic would drop to the bottom. The machine held ten different comic books, five on each side. I used my paper route money and always bought all ten. This was the one thing I enjoyed about those liquor runs with my mom. I loved those comic books and the escape they provided from the bleak situation at home.

Back then, the liquor department was separated from the rest of the store. You had to go through a turnstile to enter. They had their own cashiers as well. It was practically a store within a store. After I purchased my comic books, I pushed through the turnstile and reluctantly rejoined my mother in a liquor aisle.

Since the round trip was so long, my mother stocked up. She'd always buy a gallon of cheap Rhine wine and a couple half-gallons of vodka. Finally, she'd grab two twelve-packs of beer and ask the clerk to double-bag everything. Back then, stores used brown paper bags, which were much sturdier than the plastic bags we use today. I would end up carrying the wine and vodka, and my mom would carry the beer. Oh yeah, and her carton of cigarettes, always a carton of cigarettes. And always Salems. She only smoked Salems.

The walk back was tough, and the bags were heavy. As soon as we got home, my mother grabbed the can opener and resumed her drinking. Pop tops weren't used much until the late sixties, so dual-sided can openers were necessary drinking tools. One side would have a sharp point to punch a hole in the can, while the other was rounded and used for opening soda and beer bottles.

My mom would sit at the kitchen table, and after a few beers, she'd take the rest of it, along with the wine and vodka, and stash everything under her bed. When she was on a jag, she didn't care if the beer and wine were warm or cold. She just needed her alcohol. I would go to my room and lose myself in my comic books. My mother never did send me to a shrink. That was just the alcohol talking. At least, that's what I used to tell myself.

I reached Dr. Drexel's office. It was 11:25; I was five minutes early. I opened a door with the doctor's name emblazoned on a pane of frosted glass. The waiting room was tasteful—the walls were gray and the chairs were black leather with dark wood frames. Geometric art in primary and secondary colors adorned the walls. I approached the receptionist's desk and was greeted by an attractive young woman named Lucy.

"Good morning," she said, "may I help you?"

"Yes, hi. I have an 11:30 appointment with Dr. Drexel."

"You must be Robert." She smiled.

"Yes, I am."

She handed me a clipboard with some forms to complete. I took it and had a seat. Name, address, telephone, emergency contact. Then, a list of any medical conditions. Alcoholism was the only one that came to mind. I almost didn't list my health insurance. I didn't want anyone at Select to know I was seeing a shrink, but I knew that psychiatrists didn't come cheap, so I put down my health insurance information and returned the clipboard.

Within minutes, Lucy told me that the doctor was ready to see me, and she led me to his office. My hands were clammy, and my stomach was queasy. I studied the doctor. He was probably about 50, with neatly trimmed salt and pepper hair.

"Hello, Robert, I'm Doctor Drexel." He extended his hand.

I brushed my hands on my pants, trying to rub off the sweat. He had a firm handshake. I didn't. We entered his office, and he closed the door. The walls were gray, like the lobby, and he had a beautiful, dark mahogany desk that must have cost a fortune. His chair was also impressive—forest-green leather, with mahogany trim that matched his desk. But there was no couch. I thought there'd be a couch.

I took a seat in a nicely appointed, charcoal-colored leather chair. On the walls were a pastoral oil painting, some very nice watercolors, and his diplomas.

"So, Robert, what brings you here today?"

I had rehearsed my lines all morning, but I stumbled to find the right words. I didn't want to sound stupid. I never stopped worrying about sounding stupid.

"Well . . . um . . . I'm having a real problem with nervousness, and it seems to be getting worse. I also have a problem with alcohol. I drink too much, and my hands are always shaky."

"Do you think you're an alcoholic?"

"Yes, I believe I am."

"How often do you drink?"

"Every day. I drink every day."

"Is there a history of alcoholism in your family?"

"Yes. My mother was an alcoholic. She died almost two years ago. From cancer. She had cancer. First her colon, then it spread to her liver. But she was sober for four years before she died."

"Is your father an alcoholic?

"No. He drinks, but never to excess. He's a workaholic, but not an alcoholic. He's an attorney, and he loves his job."

We talked about my drinking at law school and my father's low opinion of me after I quit. He asked me how much I drank a day.

"Well, on workdays, I drink a six-pack of 16-ounce beers each evening. On weekends, I drink much more."

"Have you consumed any alcohol this morning?"

"No, I'm working today. I don't drink at work."

"What do you do for a living?"

"I'm a buyer at a screw and bolt company. I'm pretty much a glorified clerk."

"Would you like to quit drinking?"

"Yes, Doctor. I think I would. I feel like I'm going nowhere, and that my drinking is holding me back."

"Well, Robert. I'm inclined to agree with you. I don't think that drinking is a good choice for a lot of people."

"But when I don't drink, I'm always crazy nervous."

"Do you think the nervousness might be caused by your drinking?"

"Maybe, but all my life, even when I was a kid, I've been nervous. Nervous and shy. Timid."

"Well, Robert, I don't usually choose this route for most patients, but I think that you might benefit from taking Valium. Valium is a benzodiazepine, a sedative. I think it might be helpful."

"Is it addictive?" I asked.

"Well, addiction's a subjective term, but if you take it according to a doctor's instructions, it can be quite effective."

"I'm not sure, doctor. I don't know if I trust myself with Valium."

"I understand your reluctance, and I do have another thought. You appear to have what we call benign essential tremor. There is a medication for hypertension, high blood pressure, if you will. It's called Inderal, and it's quite effective at addressing some of your symptoms. It helps reduce shaking and jitters. This medication is a beta-blocker. Beta-blockers have been found to help with stage fright, performance anxiety, and public speaking. They can even reduce sweating."

I could not have asked for more encouraging news. Maybe I'd have a chance to stop drinking and being so anxious all the time.

"Is it addictive?" I asked again.

"No, it's not. Of course, if you are placed on a regimen of Inderal for, let's say, several weeks or months, and you want to stop, it has to be discontinued gradually. We call that titration. But as far as being addictive, that's not a concern. I would like you to try it, and if you're not happy with the results, we can revisit the Valium. How does that sound, Robert?"

"Yes, Doctor, I think I'd like to go with the Inderal."

"Okay then. I'll write you a prescription, and we'll see how things go. I'll put you on the typical starting dose, which is 80 milligrams in two divided doses. I'd like you to take 40 milligrams before dinner tonight, then another 40 milligrams tomorrow before breakfast. I'd like to see you again in four weeks, and we'll consider increasing your dose. For most essential tremor patients, the daily dose is 120 milligrams. That's 60 milligrams twice daily. Oh, I probably don't need to remind you, but it's important that you abstain from alcohol while you're taking this medication."

He handed me the prescription. I lived about two blocks from a Walgreens, so I could drop it off after work. I was feeling very hopeful.

"So, Robert, please make an appointment with Lucy on your way out, and I'll be seeing you in four weeks."

I shook his hand and left his office. I told Lucy that the doctor wanted to see me in four weeks.

"Sure thing. Four weeks from today will be Wednesday, April 6. Does that work for you?"

"April 6 is fine. May I get the 11:30 slot again?"

"Absolutely," she said, "I'll put you down for 11:30 on the sixth. Here's a card for you with the time and date."

I took the card, put it in my wallet, and smiled. "Thanks, Lucy. Have a great day."

She smiled back. "You do the same."

I walked down a flight of stairs and out of the building. That had been relatively painless. I returned to Select feeling very hopeful. I was still young—28 years old—and I had my whole life ahead of me.

When I got back to work, Dennis and Eileen asked how my appointment had gone.

"Fine," I said. I didn't elaborate.

Later, I told Rosemary about the Inderal and the tremors, and how the doctor wanted to prescribe Valium for me.

"I'm glad you said no. That's just something else to get addicted to." She knew me better than I thought.

The afternoon passed quickly, and after work, I took the Diversey bus to Broadway. I decided to walk the rest of the way home. It wasn't that far, about a mile. I reached the Walgreens and turned in my prescription at the pharmacy. A young woman told me it would be ready in a half hour, and asked if I'd like to wait. I said I would.

Twenty minutes later, she called my name and asked if I had ever taken Inderal before. When I said no, she called for a pharmacist to come to the window. He repeated everything that Dr. Drexel had told me. He poured some tablets onto a tray. They were small green hexagons with a big "I" stamped on them. They were scored on the other side, but I wouldn't need to cut them. I thanked him for his time, and the young woman rang me up.

"With your insurance, it comes to six dollars."

I paid her and was out the door. Six dollars. I thought of all the money I would save if I stopped spending half my check each week on booze. When I got home, I took my first pill. I wondered how it would make me feel. After an hour, I felt almost serene, but I knew that the real test would be riding the bus to work in the morning.

I awoke the next morning, shaved, and showered. I took my Inderal before breakfast and felt decidedly calmer on the bus ride to work. By the time I reached Select, I felt that my hands shook less, and I was more confident on the phone and with my coworkers. This medicine didn't provide the sense of bravado that only alcohol can, but I felt more settled and a lot less edgy.

I followed Dr. Drexel's instructions to lay off the alcohol, and although I missed my beer after work, I felt much better in the morning. I liked waking up sober—no more shaking, no regrets, no wondering what had happened the night before. And I could tell everyone at Select that the reason I wasn't drinking was that I was taking a blood pressure medication. I didn't have to cop to being an alcoholic, though it's not like my drinking was some closely guarded, company secret. Still, it was nice to play the blood pressure card if anyone questioned my newfound sobriety.

Friday arrived, and I enjoyed a pleasant weekend reading and exercising. Monday morning, I was walking to the main office when I ran into Ted, a nice guy who worked as an order puller in the shipping department. He was about my height, a little paunchy, and his long, rather greasy hair was turning prematurely gray.

"Hey, Rob, we missed you at Riley's on Friday."

"Hey, Ted. No more Riley's for me. The doctor put me on some blood pressure medicine, and I'm not supposed to drink with it."

"So, how long has it been since you had a drink?" he asked.

"Five days."

"Naw. You? Five days? You haven't had a single drink in five days? You're shittin' me, right?"

"No, I'm not kidding. And you know what? I like waking up without a hangover. And I can remember everything I said or did the night before."

"Wow, wait 'til I tell the other guys. They won't believe it. Rob Rickelman sober for five friggin' days. Well, I guess I oughta congratulate you."

I smiled. I felt pretty darned proud of myself as I walked to the purchasing office, feeling chipper and ready for the week ahead.

Some of my friends were skeptical of my claims of sobriety. It's funny, but when most of your friends are alcoholics, and you suddenly quit drinking, they don't know how to react. Drinking is the bond—the commonality—in these kinds of friendships. Hanging out after work, hitting the bars on Friday nights; everything revolves around drinking. So, when I decided to stop, my friends didn't know how to relate to me. At work, everyone was still friendly, but as time passed, a sense of detachment, a disconnect, developed. We were beginning to realize that without alcohol, we weren't on the same page. I knew I was better off sober, even if it meant losing my drinking buddies. As for the guys who still drank, some seemed uncomfortable around me. Maybe they wondered if they had issues with alcohol as well.

But not everyone was sorry to see me quit. Brent and Natalie were very supportive of my sobriety. And Vera in personnel now had one less drunk to worry about. Eileen was skeptical, but I think she knew I was doing the right thing. Dennis seemed curious about my decision to quit drinking. It had to be obvious to him that he was on a slippery slope.

By far, the person who was happiest about my quitting drinking was Rosemary. She had witnessed, daily, my anxiety and nervous behavior, as I watched the clock all day for work to end so I could finally have a drink. I would no longer be that person.

"Rob," she said, "I'm really proud of you. Your life will be so much better."

As for my health, I hadn't felt so good in a long time—waking up without a hangover, not afraid to start a new day. I felt refreshed, and I had gained a new sense of self-confidence. When I saw Dr. Drexel again, he seemed pleased with the results as well as my attitude. He raised my dose to 120 milligrams per day and said he'd like to see me in three months.

The next few months went well for me, but as my mind grew clearer, I realized that there was no future for me at Select. Even if Dennis left, Eileen would have a fit if I was promoted over her. I might have been okay with the title of Purchasing Director, but my role would be strictly diminished by Brent and Natalie, as well as the comptroller, Bryan. They held the real power and decision-making authority over purchasing.

In the fall of 1984, I made the boneheaded decision to leave Select and enroll at the University of Illinois at Chicago and complete my degree in political science. I needed 27 credit hours to graduate. But I could not adapt to the pressure of returning to school full-time, and I fell into my old habit of drinking before class. All the progress I'd made with the Inderal was for naught. Within a few weeks, I dropped out. I had blown my sobriety, and I was drinking every day. Again.

CHAPTER 14

Volleyball and Listerine

In the fall of 1984, after bouncing from one shitty job to another, I was once again unemployed. For some reason, probably out of pity, my father decided to take one last chance on me, and I was hired as a law clerk at the Wacker Drive law firm where he was a partner. The firm specialized in family law, which included divorce, child custody, and various disagreeable matters that arise when marriages fall apart. Family law is crazier and more hazardous than any other practice, including criminal law. People in the middle of a divorce are angry and unreasonable, and they fight viciously over their kids, their homes, their pets. They fight over everything.

My father's partner was a high-powered and extremely aggressive lawyer who flew by the seat of his pants. He made a very good living as an attorney and as a wheeler-dealer who was involved in several, often dubious, business ventures. His name was Alex Galvin, and he was a real piece of work. You couldn't help but admire him. Alex was the kind of guy you'd want on your side when the chips were down.

From my first day on the job, I had decided—once again—that I would need alcohol to deal with the stress of working in such an insane environment. I chose Listerine to boost my courage. I hoped its fragrance would be less obvious than liquors such as vodka or gin. Vodka has a reputation for being odorless, but that is a misapprehension. It smells as boozy as whiskey, beer, or any other libation. Most people don't realize it, but Listerine has an alcohol content of 26.9%, which is just about the equivalent of peppermint schnapps. I fell into a terrible routine of consuming twelve ounces of Listerine each morning before work and visiting various drugstores throughout the day to purchase smaller bottles that I drank to maintain my buzz.

I would drink a lot of beer on Fridays after work, and Saturdays from the time I woke until I passed out in the evening. I'd awaken each Sunday morning at 7:00. If I had been careful the previous day, I would have enough beer to get me through the morning. Back then, alcohol was not sold until noon on Sundays. Just knowing that I had enough handy had a calming effect, a sort of alcoholic placebo, so to speak. I never drank Listerine on the weekends; I hated its taste, but I knew that drinking it was necessary for me to do my job.

In the summer of 1985, I was part of a group that met every Sunday at Oz Park, near Halsted and Armitage, to play volleyball. There would usually be about twenty or so players, most of us in our mid-twenties and early thirties. Everyone brought their alcoholic beverage of choice. Beer was the overwhelming favorite. Booze was, for most of us—especially me—a fundamental component of the Sunday volleyball experience.

I was 30 years old and in excellent shape. I was renting a studio apartment in the old Music Box Theater building on Southport Avenue. In addition to weeknight workouts, I exercised each Sunday morning from 8:00 until 11:00. I used a bench, barbells, and dumbbells, and suffered through scores of sit-ups and push-ups. I would begin my workout after drinking a strong cup of instant coffee. At about the halfway point, I would crack open a cold beer and nurse it slowly while I continued my exercises. By the end of the session, I'd have downed two beers, hardly enough for a buzz, but adequate to get some much-needed alcohol into my system. At the end of my workout, I would treat myself to a strong screwdriver. Then, I'd brush my teeth vigorously and jump in the shower.

Once dressed, I would walk downstairs to the liquor store that was conveniently located next door. I'd purchase a twelve-pack of Old Style, return upstairs, and call a cab to get to the park. Cab fare was about three dollars, and I'd tip the driver another three. It was much cheaper than owning a car and easier than the hassle of finding a parking space.

Once I arrived, I monitored my beer intake. I knew I was a drunk, but I didn't care to advertise the fact. It's said that alcohol negatively affects one's physical skills and reflexes, but in my case, drinking was indispensable to my game. I would have been a nervous wreck without it. But with a good buzz going, I was one of the better players.

After a half-hour or so, I'd peel off my shirt. Sadly, being in shape was the only thing I had going for me. My job as a law clerk was quite a tumble from my glory days of law school. So, Sunday was my day to shine and forget about what a loser I was.

Among the regular players was a breathtakingly beautiful girl, Tricia Benjamin. Tricia was from Cleveland but worked in Chicago as an assistant for a highly regarded fashion photographer. She should have been one of the models. A friend of mine, Randy Cooper, who was also a regular, gave Tricia the perfect nickname, "Trish the Dish." I was, by every measure, smitten with her, but I was in over my head. She was fully aware of how attractive she was, and she enjoyed toying with suckers like me.

When I first met Trish, there was a mutual attraction between us. She was younger, 23 years old, and was a perfect package of feminine beauty. Trish was five foot five, about 120 pounds, and was blessed with a perfectly proportioned figure. She wore her silky, dark brown hair in a short bob with long bangs that just brushed her eyebrows. Her eyes were dark brown, and her olive skin was flawless.

We had been dating for about a month when Trish reproved me with a stinging, but deadly accurate, assessment. She said, "For someone who treats the outside of his body with so much care, you sure treat your insides like shit."

She was making the obvious point that I drank too much. When the relationship was just about over, I called her and asked if we could meet somewhere and talk. She said, "We could meet for coffee. Wait, that won't work, will it? You'd need to meet for cocktails."

I never saw her again. I kept going to volleyball, but she stayed away. She wanted nothing more to do with me. This hurt something fierce, but I couldn't blame her.

Once Trish stopped showing up for volleyball, I was much less careful about hiding my drinking. When the games ended, I would head to Glascott's, a popular bar, and quaff several pints of Guinness.

After an hour, I would leave Glascott's and hail a cab home, arriving, very drunk, around 7:00. I'd hit the fridge for one last beer, then pass out.

Six o'clock on Monday was signaled by the headache-inducing beep of my alarm clock. I'd awaken, miserably hungover, with the shakes about to set in. I'd drink a glass of cold water to wake myself up. Then, I would go to the closet to retrieve a large bottle of Listerine.

The first swig was so foul that it was impossible to keep down.

My normal routine involved belting down a slug, which almost immediately came back up, scorching both my nostrils and throat. That shit was hell in a bottle. The trick was to take small sips, then puke. I'd repeat this procedure until enough alcohol accumulated in my gut to stop the heaving and the shakes. After the buzz sank in, it didn't taste so revolting.

I followed this up with a thorough tooth brushing, a shave, and a hot shower. Once out of the shower, I would drink about 12 more ounces and dress for work. I chewed bubble gum to mask the odor and walked three blocks to the "L" station. I'd arrive at work at 8:45 and check in with my dad and the secretaries. And I would take the daily morning phone call from Alex with his long list of assignments. Among them were going to court to file motions, hitting the county clerk's office for more filing, and making deliveries to various law offices.

After a few hours, my Listerine buzz would wane, so I would duck into a Walgreens to buy a three or six-ounce bottle that I would down in the nearest public restroom.

I spent most afternoons in the office, doing research, once in a while interviewing clients, and often helping my favorite secretary, Tanya, decipher the convoluted Dictaphone messages that Alex would leave for her. Tanya was a very attractive, African-American, single mother of a seven-year-old boy, and she had a lovely personality. I was quite fond of her, and we worked well together. I was pretty sure she knew about the drinking, but she never said a word about it.

Finally, after making it through another day, I would leave work and head to a liquor store to purchase a half-pint of genuine peppermint schnapps. I'd drop into either the Daley Center or the State of Illinois building, both of which had several public restrooms, and savor my schnapps. Compared to Listerine, it was top shelf.

I'd arrive home by 7:30, drink another beer, eat two cold hot dogs from the fridge, and hit the sack. The next morning, I would suffer through my scheduled bout with the Listerine.

This was the drill from Monday through Thursday. On Fridays, I would still drink the schnapps, but I would ride the "L" train to a stop on the Northside where I would visit Berlin, a bar that featured the best new-wave music videos and a fascinating mix of gay and straight clientele. I never looked for anyone to hook up with. I was there to relax and unwind, and to mark the conclusion of another dreadful week of work.

CHAPTER 15

Unauthorized Practice of Law

In late 1985, my father and Joanne, one of our secretaries, with whom he was having an affair, moved to San Diego. He didn't even bother to divorce his second wife, Coralee, until many years later. After they left, Ellen Burke became Alex's partner. She was a good lawyer and easy to work for. My responsibilities at the office increased significantly, as did my Listerine intake.

Alex was always incredibly busy, and he saved time by assigning me several extra responsibilities. One assignment that I'll never forget involved an extraordinarily beautiful client.

On a pleasant Thursday morning in late April of 1986, I arrived for work at my typical time, 8:45. I was in the office preparing for a busy morning at the Daley Center Courthouse. At about 8:50, Alex called the office. He was running late, as usual, and had just left his house in the upscale North Shore suburb of Highland Park. He was calling from his car.

A car phone was a rare extravagance in 1986, but Alex always owned the best of everything. By today's standards, these phones were jumbo-sized, and most required being hooked up to some sort of power source, such as a car's cigarette lighter. But his phone was, by 1980s standards, quite sleek. This Motorola model was about ten inches high, weighed about two pounds, and was equipped with a long, flexible, rubber antenna. They were often referred to as "brick phones," which was a fairly accurate description. But these bricks were among the first "car" phones that you could use when you were away from your vehicle. They were very cool. And expensive, with a price tag of about $4000.

Deborah, the receptionist, handed me the phone. "It's Alex. He wants to talk to you."

Alex drove an amazing, midnight-blue, 1986 Mercedes 560SEC. It was powered by a 5.5-liter V8 with a four-speed automatic transmission. That was fortunate because I sucked at driving a stick shift. I loved that car and took great joy in piloting it, which I did when tasked with locating and serving individuals with legal papers—subpoenas, summonses, and the like. I loved that part of my job, and I was damn good at it. I was far more efficient than the county sheriffs, who had no stake in tracking their quarry and put little effort into finding them.

I took the phone.

"Hey, Rob," Alex said, "I'm running real late, so I need you to meet a client at the courthouse on South Michigan. Tell her I'm running late, but I'll get there.

"What's her name?" I asked.

"Darcy Peterson. She's a fucking doll. Five-foot-five, great body, brown, shoulder-length hair. She'll be wearing a charcoal-gray dress, and she'll be waiting just outside the courthouse. I described you to her. I said you could pass for Richard Gere's twin brother. Take her to Judge Sandberg's courtroom, and if they call her case, tell the judge I'm on my way."

That didn't sound too difficult.

Suddenly, over the phone, I heard a loud bang.

"Jesus! I just crashed my fucking car. Damn, fucking shit."

"Are you okay?" I asked.

"Yeah, I'm fine. I wasn't paying attention to traffic. The fucking car is probably totaled. I'm gonna try to pull over."

My heart sank. I have to admit that I was more worried about the car than I was about Alex. His ethics were starting to rub off on me, and he might have approved. I could hear the sounds of the highway—cars and trucks whizzing by. Finally, Alex came back to the phone.

"All right. I'm gonna have to get this thing towed. I gotta take a cab. So, we're gonna have to change our plans. When they call the case, you're going to approach the bench like you're a lawyer. Introduce yourself, state your name, tell the judge you're from our firm, but don't say you're a fucking lawyer. Tell him you're there to get a Rule to Show Cause against the ex-husband, Gregory Peterson. He's a fucking scumbag who's been jacking Darcy around and withholding child support. Her file is on the couch in my office. I know you've never done this kind of thing before, but it's a piece of cake.

"Then you'll have to elicit some testimony from Darcy. Simple shit. Her name, divorce date, order for support, and how much he's in arrears. Then ask the judge for a rule, write it up, and you're out of there. Easy, right?"

What the fuck? He wanted me to pretend to be a lawyer in front of a fucking judge. What was that? A felony? A misdemeanor? I didn't know, but I knew I was screwed if I got caught.

I laughed nervously.

"Just have fun with it. I promise you, she's a babe. I've got faith in you. Now I've gotta get this fucking wreck taken care of. Put Deborah back on."

I handed the phone to Deborah and went into Alex's office to get the file. What a fucking mess. His desk was buried in files, and others lay all over the floor, but I found Darcy's file on the couch where he said it would be. Even with all the Listerine I'd consumed, my stomach was churning like crazy. I was so fucking nervous.

I grabbed the file, said goodbye to Deborah, and took the elevator to the lobby. I stopped at a Walgreens, bought a six-ounce bottle of Listerine, and ducked into an alley. This was pretty risky—I preferred the privacy of a restroom—but I was in a hurry. I drank the whole thing in about half a minute. I threw the empty into a dumpster, headed to State Street, and grabbed a cab to the courthouse.

When we arrived, I exited the cab and spotted a lovely young woman waiting near the entrance. Alex Galvin was inclined to exaggerate, but this time, he had understated just how gorgeous Darcy Peterson was. As soon as I saw her, my hands grew damp and sweaty. It was bad enough trying to pass myself off as a lawyer, but to do so in the presence of such a striking beauty was beyond my ken.

I approached her.

"Are you Darcy Peterson?" I asked.

"Yes. You work for Alex?"

I extended a clammy hand. "Yes. I'm Rob Rickelman. I have some news for you. Alex totaled his car and won't be able to make it this morning. I have your file, and I'm going to represent you." I decided not to tell her that I wasn't an attorney. This was going to be an ordeal, and I was already overwhelmed.

"Well, let's get this over with," she said.

We walked together up the steps and through the metal detectors. I tried to avoid breathing Listerine in her face.

"The hearing is in Judge Sandberg's courtroom. Here it is," I said.

We entered and took our seats in the front row, just behind the attorneys' tables. The judge was not on the bench yet. I checked my watch. It was 9:20. The docket call was ten minutes away. I didn't know what to say to this beautiful young woman, so I busied myself reviewing the case files. Darcy sat silently. I hoped she couldn't smell my breath.

I had the papers that Tanya had prepared for me. I was to present a motion for a Rule to Show Cause why the respondent should not be held in contempt of court for failing to pay child support and for failing to appear as ordered. In family court, the defendant was called the respondent, and the plaintiff was the petitioner. Darcy was the petitioner. I had a pretty good handle on the nuances of family court, but I was terrified of speaking before the judge and in the middle of a crowded courtroom.

It was almost 9:30. I wanted to get this over with as quickly as possible. I wished I could sneak into the restroom and guzzle some more Listerine, but that wasn't going to happen.

At 9:30 sharp, a short, stocky bailiff wearing a starched white shirt and navy-blue slacks entered the courtroom through a door on the right side of the bench. In a booming, officious voice, he announced, "All rise. The First Municipal Court of Cook County, Family Division, the Honorable Peter Sandberg presiding, is now in session."

I was immediately swept by a strong wave of nausea. *"Oh, God, don't let me puke,"* I prayed.

The bailiff was followed by the judge, a tall, handsome, and distinguished gentleman with a full head of snowy white hair. He perfectly fit the image of a stately, refined, and learned jurist. He took his seat behind the bench and said, "Good morning, everyone. Please be seated."

The court clerk, a short, chubby woman with large, clear,

plastic-framed glasses, sat at the left side of the bench. Her seat and desk were situated a few feet below the judge, who was provided a vantage point above the rest of us.

The clerk called the first case, which, unfortunately, was not ours. But we didn't have to wait long. At 9:50, she called our case, "Peterson v. Peterson," and Darcy and I hurriedly rose.

I nervously said, "Petitioner Darcy Peterson is present, Your Honor."

My heart was thumping, my throat was parched, and my hands were moist and shaky. I was careful not to identify myself as "counsel for the petitioner."

We stepped before the judge, and I said, "Good morning, Your Honor. Robert Rickelman, from Galvin and Burke, on behalf of the petitioner, Darcy Peterson."

The judge nodded. So far, so good. I knew that he was well-acquainted with my father, who had been before him dozens of times. My father had a deep respect for Judge Sandberg. I was hoping he wouldn't mention my dad or ask me when I had passed the bar, which of course, had never fucking happened. I was treading on very thin ice.

The judge looked at the papers his clerk had handed him.

"Good morning, Counsel. Is the respondent present?"

Counsel, he called me Counsel.

I looked at the crowd and was relieved that no one else was approaching.

"The respondent isn't in the courtroom, Your Honor. In fact, Mr. Peterson has been absent for the last three hearings, although his attorney, Dennis Field, has received notice to appear prior to each court date."

"So, you're seeking a Rule to Show Cause this morning?"

"Yes, we are, Your Honor."

"Is the petitioner prepared to go forward?"

"Yes, Judge, she is."

"Okay then, Counsel, you may proceed."

This was my cue to "elicit testimony" from our client. The bailiff swore her in. I took a deep breath and turned toward her.

"Would you state your name for the record, please?"

"Darcy Peterson," she said.

I thought my head was going to explode. I fought to steady myself. How the fuck had I ended up here? Mother-fucking Alex, that's how.

Throughout our line of questioning, we established that Darcy and her husband had two kids, and he was in arrears for over half a year. She also testified that this was the fourth time he hadn't shown up for court.

I turned toward the judge. "Your Honor, at this time, petitioner, Darcy Peterson, is seeking a Rule to Show Cause why respondent, Gregory Peterson, should not be held in contempt of this Court for failing to appear on, including today, four occasions."

The judge said, "The Court finds that such rule should issue to the effect that respondent, Gregory Peterson, is to appear on May 5 to give reason why he should not be held in contempt of court. Counsel, draft the order. And, oh yes. Please say hello to your father. I understand he's living the good life in San Diego."

My heart jerked when he said that. "Thank you, Judge," I said. "I'll do that. Have a good morning, Your Honor."

I whispered for Darcy to take a seat while I went to one of the long attorneys' tables to draft the order and have it entered by the clerk. The clerk gave me my copies. They were still using carbon paper back then.

I breathed a long sigh of relief. The entire courtroom probably reeked of Listerine, but I had done it. I had walked into court, presented myself before the judge, and gotten a court order for a very beautiful, though very unimpressed, client.

I thought about Darcy's ex. Man, how could he blow it with a creature as beautiful as she was? Well, she wasn't the nicest person, that was for sure.

Darcy and I left the courthouse, and I walked her to her car.

"Well," I said, "that's it until May."

"Tell Alex to call me. Today."

She walked to her car without thanking me. But that didn't matter. I was a drunk, no doubt about it. But that day, I was a drunk who had rolled the dice and won. I had done what very few people would have risked, and I'd done it well. Alex would be pleased.

I hailed a cab and headed back to the office. I exited the taxi and stopped at a Walgreens for a six-ouncer of Listerine. I ducked into the Daley Center, found a restroom, and toasted my victory. Extralegal or not, it was mine to enjoy.

CHAPTER 16

A Wrong Move to San Diego

Everywhere I went, and everything I did at Galvin and Burke, required a bellyful of Listerine. My eyes were always glassy and bloodshot. I tried all the eye-drop brands, but nothing got the red out.

Mandy Norwood was the secretary who replaced Joanne when she left with my father. Mandy was very bossy. I did not like her, and I did not let her tell me what to do. One morning, she came into my office and started badgering me about some papers I had forgotten to file at the county clerk's office. I was in no mood to be yelled at by this self-important witch.

"Shut the fuck up!" I yelled.

And off she went. "Your daddy's not here anymore, so you better learn your place. You're a clerk here, and I'm a legal secretary. Don't you ever dare talk to me like that again."

She was so mad she was shaking. If it weren't for my Listerine buzz, I'd be shaking too. I was furious and I lost it.

"Get the hell out of my office. You're not my fucking boss."

"We're not through, you disrespectful little jerk," she said as she stormed away.

She was gone, but she wanted to even the score. The next morning, after Alex, Ellen, and the rest of us had finished the morning court rush, Ellen called me into her office. I had a sneaking suspicion of what we'd be discussing.

Her door was closed. I knocked, and she told me to come in.

"Hi, Rob. Have a seat."

I sat in a chair next to her desk.

"This is hard to say, but Alex wanted me to talk to you."

"I think I know why," I said. I was riding a wave of nausea.

"Rob, it's pretty obvious to everyone that you've been drinking at work. You know, we really can't have anyone drinking on the job."

"I don't know what to say. You're right. My drinking is inexcusable," I said. I knew it was just a matter of time until someone called me out on it.

"You know, Rob, I experienced a drinking problem a few years back. It got pretty bad. I never drank at work, but I drank every night. A lot. So, I saw a shrink for a while and was totally abstinent for almost a year. Now, I drink once in a while. Only socially and on some weekends. You can beat this thing. You just have to make up your mind. Alex is willing to pay for you to go to rehab."

She didn't know about my rehab in 1981.

"Thanks, Ellen, but I just don't think I can quit drinking."

"Would you like to try?"

"To tell you the truth, I don't know. I'm not sure I could do this job, all this stuff, you know, without drinking."

"You're an extremely bright guy, and you have a great disposition. Everyone here really likes you."

"Everyone but Mandy," I said.

"Let's not focus on Mandy right now. This is about you. We want to help, Alex and I. You owe it to yourself to try. You don't need the alcohol, believe me."

"I have to tell you, Ellen. I was in rehab a few years back, and when I got out, I didn't stay sober for a week. I don't want to go back to rehab."

"Well, if you won't go to rehab, Alex wants you to take some time off. You have one week's pay for last week, and he wants to pay you an extra two weeks. Call it vacation pay. That's three weeks total. When you're clean and feeling better, maybe we can talk about your coming back to work."

"Thanks, Ellen. I think I'd like to try that route."

"Okay. Alex didn't think you'd go for the rehab, so I'm going to write you a check for $1200."

I couldn't believe my good luck. Ellen was being very nice, and $1200 would last me until I dried myself out or got some shitty warehouse job where I could drink on the sly. My rent and utilities were pretty cheap, about $400 a month. I could make this money last before I had to find another job.

"Thanks, Ellen. I'll take the check and work on drying out." I wanted that check in my hands, and I wanted out of there.

Ellen wrote the check and handed it to me. I had to get out of there. I quickly shook her hand, made a beeline past Deborah, and pressed the elevator button. I got downstairs and headed to the bank to cash the check. I had $1200 in my pocket. It had been a very long time since I'd had that much cash. I wanted to duck into the nearest bar and celebrate my freedom. Freedom from Alex, freedom from Mandy, and freedom from Listerine. I felt that a heavy weight had been lifted off my chest.

It's funny how quickly life can change. A few weeks earlier, Alex had offered to pay me $12 an hour, and more incredibly, he offered to pay my law school tuition. I knew it wasn't a good idea to accept his generous offer. I imagined the kind of mischief

I would be involved in if I did finish law school and went to work for Alex. As things turned out, Alex eventually lost his license to practice and was permanently disbarred a few years later.

The bar I chose was just opening for lunch. I ordered a shot of Jack Daniel's and a beer. Ten minutes later, I was out the door and headed to the "L." I stopped at the liquor store for some more booze. Vodka and beer were what I needed, and I was going to enjoy the hell out of them.

I liked my small apartment, the neighborhood was decent, and a trend toward gentrification had already begun. I holed up in my studio apartment, leaving only to stock up on booze at the liquor store next door or the Jewel Supermarket across the street to buy food. I wasn't eating very much, but I was drinking heavily. It didn't take long before the severance money I'd received was running low, and I was in no condition to start looking for a job. I needed my alcohol—I could not imagine being without it.

Somehow, my father caught wind of the fact that I was no longer working at Galvin and Burke, so he arranged for Kevin to fly in from San Diego to convince me to move to my dad's and Joanne's house in La Mesa. Kevin, Kerry, and Kathy were also living with them, as well as Joanne's young son, Logan.

My phone rang continuously, but I never answered it. Kevin and Kurt were leaving messages for me, telling me that they wanted to talk to me about moving to California. They said my airfare would be taken care of, and that I could live rent-free at my dad's house until I got back on my feet. I did not want my family to see me drunk, or worse, in the throes of withdrawal. And, the bottom line was that I didn't want to stop drinking.

I knew that it was only a matter of time before my brothers paid me a visit. One Friday night, June 6, there was a knock on my door. It was 11:00, and I could hear Kurt and Kevin calling my name. They had talked the manager, Santiago, into unlocking my door so they could see if I was in there. I had anticipated they might be allowed to enter, so I crawled into the tiny cabinet under the kitchen sink. I could barely close the door, but I fit snugly inside. After my brothers left, I thought I was good until daybreak, but at about 1:00 a.m., they paid me a second visit and found me passed out on my bed. I'd had a good run.

Kevin and I spent the weekend at Kurt's and his girlfriend's house in Oak Park. They weren't letting me out of their sight. I was able to convince them to allow me my beer and vodka, which I tried to drink in moderation. Saturday morning, I woke at 6:00, and while Kurt and Kevin were still asleep, I helped myself to a good deal of alcohol.

At 8:00 on Sunday morning, June 8, I placed two suitcases stuffed with clothes into the trunk of Kevin's rental car. We said our goodbyes to Kurt and drove to O'Hare Airport for a 10:00 flight to San Diego. Once we were airborne, the flight attendant came to offer sodas and juice. I asked her for a gin and tonic; it cost $4.00. Before we laid over in Denver, I ordered a second drink.

We landed at Stapleton Airport at noon Mountain Time. We would be changing planes, and I convinced Kevin to accompany me to a bar near our gate. I ordered a bottle of Coors, and Kevin did as well. I slugged mine down while Kevin nursed his. I ordered one more beer before we boarded our flight.

After takeoff, I waited for the beverage cart and ordered another gin and tonic. Kevin asked for a Heineken. I gave the flight attendant $8.00, and before we reached San Diego, I ordered one last drink. By the time we landed, I felt sufficiently buzzed to greet my father and Joanne, who met us at the baggage carousel. I was sure my father could tell I had been drinking, but he didn't say anything. Not until we arrived at his house. He then made it clear that my staying there was contingent on my absolute abstinence from any sort of liquor. For the next few days, I stayed in my bedroom to dry out. The withdrawal from booze, as always, was a mother fucker.

It didn't take long for me to realize what a terrible mistake I had made in moving to San Diego and into a large house with my father, his girlfriend, and her son. Kevin had a great job as a wine salesman, and he drove a brand-new car, a blue 1986 Mazda 626. I loved that car. He was living the good life; I envied him but was happy that he was doing well. Kerry and Kathy were also doing fine, and Kevin's girlfriend, Cheryl, had a good job too.

Within a few months, I resumed my drinking and had a huge falling out with my father and Joanne. I called my father a fucking prick, and Joanne accurately called me an ass-hole drunk. My father told me that if I didn't leave immediately, he would call the police. So, I packed a few things and was out the door for good.

CHAPTER 17

Phyllis

After the *desmadre* with my father and Joanne, I once again had no place to live. My brother Kerry had a friend, Gilbert, who allowed me to sleep on his couch, provided I stayed off the sauce.

I moved in on Thursday, November 20, 1986. Within two days, I'd finished all of Gilbert's alcohol, which consisted of a full fifth of vodka and a liter of what turned out to be some very expensive tequila.

On Saturday morning, I was confronted by a very angry Gilbert and told that I had half an hour to pack my things. I called Kevin and asked him to help me out. Again.

Kevin picked me up at noon. He said he didn't have much money, and I didn't blame him for his reluctance to front me any cash. But he didn't know what else to do with me. Against his better judgment, he agreed to lend me three hundred dollars. I swore up and down that I would use the money for food and rent only, and I would not use it to buy alcohol. Kevin wasn't an idiot, and I knew he didn't believe me, but he was giving me one last chance to do the right thing. He let me know that this would be the last money he would give me, and I knew I'd have to find a job quickly. Before the money ran out.

As far as my accommodations, Kevin suggested the seedy

Gaslamp area, which was just south of downtown San Diego and within our budget. We drove to the Gaslamp, and there was no shortage of run-down SROs. I looked out the window, surveying the denizens of this bleak, decaying neighborhood. There were drunks, hookers, and a handful of disabled vets flying their cardboard signs, asking for handouts, spare change, and the like. These were my brethren. It was hard to imagine a more dreary setting.

The hotels, in their sorry condition, reminded me of my time at the Maybrook, where I spent several alcohol-soaked months. I missed the short period after I moved out of the Maybrook when I strung together a few months of quality sobriety. But I could not stay sober anymore.

Kevin found a parking space in front of a drab, gray, three-story building, the Prince Albert. It had probably once been a nice place, but that would have been many years ago.

While Kevin waited in the car, I got out and walked up the steps of the hotel and through the main entrance. There were two steel doors on either side of the small foyer, probably one for the boiler room, and the other, perhaps a supply room. The front desk was one floor up. I opened a second door and walked quickly upstairs. I didn't want to keep Kevin waiting.

Once upstairs, I approached the front desk clerk. He was a big, bald-headed guy in a dirty white T-shirt that not only highlighted his full, round belly but also accentuated some exceptionally large biceps. He was a very intimidating, no-nonsense guy. And, he needed a shave.

I hadn't had a drink since the day before, and I was extremely anxious. I wished I could have had a few drinks to help me get through this. But Kevin had refused to stop and buy me any booze. I'd have to do this sober. Sober and shaky. The clerk, whose name was Frank, told me that a week's rent was $60, and was expected on time, every Saturday, by noon—no exceptions, no excuses, no charity.

I told Frank that I'd be right back and ran downstairs to get the money from Kevin. This would pay the rent for a few weeks and leave me some cash for food and liquor. I could not imagine living in this flophouse without a good, strong buzz.

I thanked Kevin, grabbed my things, and rushed upstairs to pay Frank my first week's rent. He gave me my key and pointed out my room, number 21. *Shit*, I thought, *I'm only a few doors from the desk.* Then, I reasoned that being near the front desk might mean less noise and a better night's sleep.

After I checked in, I went to my room. It was more dismal than the Maybrook. Everything was dingy and smoke-covered, and the bed was a twin-size with a rusty metal frame and a thin, worn-out mattress.

Against the wall were an old wooden desk and a rickety chair with dirty, tattered, orange upholstery. The sink had two faucets—one hot, the other cold, just as at the Maybrook. And, just as at the Maybrook, this sink would double as my urinal.

I walked down the hall to check the men's bathroom; it was moldy, smelly, and disgusting. Someone must have taken a nasty shit just before I walked in. I tried to hold my breath. But I had to stay positive. I would get a job and move out of this dump as soon as I could. For now, though, with Kevin gone, it was time to get some alcohol. So, I left my second-floor hovel in search of a cheap liquor store.

I found a place that catered to winos. That meant they sold fortified, or screw-cap wine, better known as bum wine, with catchy names like Mad Dog, Thunderbird, and Night Train. They also carried a selection of 40-ounce bottles of malt liquor, which contained much more alcohol than regular beer. I bought a forty-ouncer, an eighteen-pack of cheap beer, and two fifths of low-end vodka. It was probably one rung above rubbing alcohol.

The liquor store also sold ramen noodles for 50¢ a package, which was a rip-off. I had no stove, so I would sprinkle the seasoning on the noodles and eat them dry. They tasted pretty good that way. I bought four packs of ramen and headed back to the hotel.

As I passed the front desk, I wondered if Frank noticed, or even cared, about the eighteen-pack and the heavy brown grocery bag I was carrying.

I estimated that the alcohol I'd bought would be enough to last me three or four days, as long as I didn't get crazy and drink it all up. I would have to conserve, drinking just enough to keep my head straight and my courage high. Monday morning, I'd start my job search.

I didn't want to waste my money on the price of a Sunday paper, so I'd find a library. For the time being, I steadied my nerves with some stiff drinks.

I quickly drank two cans of beer, then poured a few ounces of warm vodka into a glass. The vodka burned when I swallowed it; I needed the buzz and savored the burn. I lay down on the bed and looked at my watch. It was 3:00 p.m., November 22, 1986, the start of my exciting new life in downtown San Diego. I thought to myself that Thanksgiving was less than a week away. But that year, it would merely be another date on the calendar. I opened the forty-ouncer, emptied it within twenty minutes, and dozed off.

When I awoke, the room was dark. There was some faint light filtering in from the parking lot next door. It was just after midnight. I drank a beer, poured myself some vodka, and went back to sleep.

I woke up Sunday morning at 6:15. The sun hadn't fully risen, and the room was still dark. It was time for a beer. I popped one open and drank it quickly. I was surprised to have acquired a strange craving for an orange soda. There was a vending machine near the front entrance, but I'd need a few ounces of vodka before I could leave my room. I poured half a glass and drained it.

The vodka seared my throat, so I cupped my hand and drank some tepid water from the cold-water faucet. I sat on the bed, relishing the early morning buzz that warmed my gut and soothed my soul.

Feeling sufficiently composed, I opened my door and was surprised to see a young woman, petite, probably Hispanic, and very pretty. She had coal-black eyes that matched her raven-dark, shoulder-length hair. Her bangs were short as if she'd cut them herself. But the short bangs accentuated her lovely olive skin. She wore a yellow cotton halter, white shorts that showed a lot of leg, and a pair of pink, rubber thong sandals. She was exquisite, but she looked exhausted. Not so much a lack of sleep tired; more a world-weary languid.

Then, there were the bruises. Her arms and legs bore several painful-looking red and purple blotches. She even had one on her face, high on her forehead, partially hidden by her bangs. I didn't know much about HIV or AIDS, but that's what I figured was the reason for so many patches of discolored skin.

She met my gaze and smiled. "Good morning, you must be new here." She had probably just finished working the street.

I smiled. "Good morning. Yeah, you're right, I just moved in yesterday." I tried to act as sober as possible, and by my standards, I wasn't all that drunk.

"Well, hi, I'm Phyllis. I've been here since June."

I did some quick math and reckoned that she had been living there for five months. Nearly half a year in this fucking dump.

"Hi, Phyllis. I'm Rob. Pleased to meet you."

Phyllis had a sweet disposition that made me instantly fond of her. "So, Rob, what brings you to the luxurious Prince Albert Hotel?"

"I'm here for the ambiance." I grinned nervously. Boy, that was lame. "Umm, actually, I'm a little tight on funds," I said.

"Don't I know it. Well, this place isn't as bad as it looks. There are three desk clerks; Dora and Alfredo are real nice. I guess you met Frank yesterday. He's a big asshole. And he doesn't take any shit, especially when the rent's due. He doesn't cut anyone any slack. Just a reminder, ya know?"

"Yeah, thanks. You're right. He wasn't all that charming when I checked in."

Phyllis laughed. "Charming? Nope, charming is definitely not a word I would use to describe Frank."

"Well, I'm heading downstairs to get a can of pop," I said.

"Pop, hunh? Chicago?"

"Yeah, I guess I mean soda."

"No, I like the way you Chicago people say pop."

"Where are you from?" I asked.

"San Diego, born and raised. Local kid makes good."

She smiled wanly. It was a joke, but it wasn't funny. She didn't mean it to be funny.

"Well . . . um . . . can I get you anything? A soda?"

"Yeah, ya know, a Dr. Pepper would hit the spot. Here's a buck. The machine is 50¢, use the change to get yourself one."

"Thanks, but you don't have to do that."

"Hey, you're doing me a favor. I want to do a favor for you."

"Thanks, I'll be right back."

As I headed downstairs, I couldn't take my mind off the lesions. I wondered if she was dying. AIDs was a formidable disease in the '80s, and to my untrained eye, her case looked fairly well advanced.

I wondered how her customers, her Johns, could overlook her very obvious bruising. Were they that desperate to get laid?

I walked to the corner and stopped at the soda machine. It was bolted to the pavement and was equipped with an iron cage to deter theft. I put in a dollar bill and pressed Dr. Pepper. A can dropped down the chute, and two quarters fell into the change holder. I put them into the coin slot, pressed Orange Crush, and my can came down with a thud. I walked back upstairs. Phyllis was still there, smoking a cigarette. A Marlboro. She offered me one.

"No, thanks. Smoking's probably the one bad habit I don't have." I handed her the Dr. Pepper.

"Bad habit? Gee, thanks."

I blushed. I appreciated her sense of humor. She was sweet, but I'm sure she had to be pretty fucking tough to turn tricks in this rundown area, or anywhere for that matter.

"Yeah, I can thank my dad for that," I said. "When I was twelve, my nine-year-old brother and I asked him if we could smoke some cigars. He said sure, under one condition: Once Keith, my brother, and I lit our cigars, we had to smoke the whole things.

"We couldn't believe that our dad had said yes. So we rushed to the corner store and bought two Parodi cigars. I think we paid a buck for the two of them. They looked like stubby little Slim Jims.

"We were back home in no time. Our dad told us to smoke them in the backyard. He didn't want us smelling up the house with cigar smoke. He lit them for us, and we started puffing away. We inhaled them like we'd seen our mom do when she smoked her cigarettes. We didn't know you weren't supposed to inhale cigars.

"Our dad chuckled and said, 'Enjoy yourselves. Let me know when you're finished.'

"We didn't even get halfway through, and we were both puking our guts out. Our dad heard the noise and came outside.

"'You haven't finished your cigars, guys. Is there a problem?'

"'Please, Dad. We're so sick. Can't we stop?'

"'Okay, here's the deal. You can stop smoking, but I don't ever want you to see you smoking anything again. Cigars, pipes, cigarettes. Nothing.'

"'Okay, Dad,' we promised in the middle of our heaving."

"'Stay out here until you feel better. Do your puking outside.'

"Then he walked into the house laughing. But you know what? That killed the smoking bug for me . . . well . . . until pot."

"And your brother?"

"You know what? He smokes cigars and a pipe. He's a better man than I am."

She laughed. I hoped I'd cheered her up. "Well, Mr. Parodi, that was quite a tale. Now I've got to get some sleep. Thanks for the pop."

"Soda," I corrected her.

Phyllis laughed. "Soda."

I hoped she wasn't dying.

CHAPTER 18

Leaving Prince Albert

I awoke at 5:00 a.m., Sunday, December 14. I did not have the sixty dollars to pay for another week at the Prince Albert and would have to be gone soon. The rent was due each Saturday, but I had asked the desk clerk, Dora, who was very sweet, if I could pay it a day late. I made up some bullshit about my brother showing up Sunday morning to front me the rent money. That was not going to happen, and I needed to get the hell out of there before Frank caught wind of my lie.

I poured myself a tumbler of vodka, which I grasped with two trembling hands so it wouldn't spill. I downed it all and lay back, waiting for a sense of peace to descend on me. It didn't take long until my jangled nerves had settled. I decided to have a final shower and shave. The lobby and hallway were empty. I walked the short distance to the bathroom, shaved quickly, showered in the grimy, foul-smelling stall, and returned to my room.

Being well-scrubbed and clean-shaven cheered me a bit. I filled another glass, which I was able to hold with one hand. The shakes were gone for the time being, but I knew they'd be back with a vengeance when the alcohol ran out. It was almost six. I was about to join the ranks of San Diego's homeless population. I was 31 years old, underweight, frail, and not cut out for that kind of life.

I still had an unopened fifth of vodka and most of a pint. I downed a bit more and prepared to leave. I stuffed the bottles into a small nylon bag with a few T-shirts, socks, and underwear. I wished I had some warmer clothes, but I hadn't anticipated ending up on the streets.

I put an ear to the door, listening carefully, trying to determine if anyone was working the desk, but I couldn't hear anything. I opened the door and made a beeline for the exit. I didn't even see if anyone was behind the desk. I rushed down the stairs and onto the street. No one followed me.

It was a wonderful morning, about 60 degrees. The sky was clear, and the sun shone brightly. This was the kind of weather that brought tourists to San Diego in the winter. I took a deep breath and counted my blessings.

The neighborhood had been run into the ground long ago. Because it was a Sunday, I passed only homeless people and drifters, each a grimier version of myself. As I roamed the neighborhood, I spotted a small grocery store. I entered the shop and bought a can of Spam. I asked the clerk for a plastic spoon, and he obliged me. I would save the Spam for dinner. I counted the change, which didn't take long. Seventy-five cents. That wouldn't buy much.

I wandered amid the dreary surroundings. It was approaching noon. I figured that the Greyhound Station might be a suitable place for me to hang out, try to be invisible. I reached the station and proceeded to the restroom. I ducked into a stall, latched the door, unzipped my bag, and retrieved the pint. I finished the bottle, knowing that I would need a considerable buzz to get through my first day and night without a roof over my head. I still had the full fifth, which I didn't open.

Feeling fortified, I left the restroom and found a seat in the waiting area. I tried not to draw any attention to myself. My clothes were clean, and I hadn't yet acquired the disheveled look of a homeless person. But within a few minutes, a security guard asked to see my ticket. Since I had nothing to show, I was told to leave.

I walked and walked, and by 5:00 p.m., it was growing dark. With the sun setting, the temperature dropped quickly. I dreaded the long night ahead. I trudged up and down Broadway, trying in vain to stay warm, but the cold was getting the best of me.

At about seven, I spotted a small crowd milling around outside the bus station. A man and woman, probably in their mid-thirties, approached me, and the man struck up a conversation.

"It's gonna be a cold one tonight."

"Yup," I answered.

"Don't you have a coat or something warm to wear?"

"I'm counting on the vodka to keep me warm."

"Vodka? What? Are you an alcoholic or something?"

"Yeah, I am. No way I could do this without the booze."

"Me and the wife never touch the stuff. So, you drink every day or what?"

He continued. "Alcohol affects your judgment," he said. "You have to have your wits about you to live on the streets."

"I'll take my chances," I said as I walked away.

People came and went. Around ten, a police cruiser rolled by, and a cop told us that we were in a no-loitering zone, so get moving. I didn't know where to go, but I left the station. I thought of letting the cops arrest me. At least a jail cell would be warm. But I did not want to lose my vodka and quickly dismissed that notion.

I ducked behind a garbage dumpster, pulled out the fifth, and guzzled some. I screwed the cap back on and found a bus stop bench. I was very hungry. I opened my bag and retrieved my can of Spam. The metal lid reminded me of the top of a sardine can.

I opened the lid and peeled it off. Above the meat was a layer of a cold, gooey gelatinous substance. I was so hungry that I scooped it up and ate it. It was surprisingly tasty. Once I'd cleaned the gooey layer, the meat didn't look half bad. I was famished and ready to eat.

As I was about to dig in, I was approached by a tough-looking guy, about my height, six feet, give or take, wearing a dirty green army jacket and a ratty pair of jeans. He had a thick neck, a sturdy jaw, and a nose that looked like it had been broken more than a few times. I was unnerved by his presence, and I knew what he wanted.

"Hey, man, I sure could use some of that Spam," he said.

"Sorry, this is lunch and dinner. I don't have any extra."

"C'mon, bro. I am starving. I haven't eaten in two days. Can't you share a little taste?"

I was glad to have the vodka in my belly. It gave me the courage to deal with this guy.

"I can't," I said. " I barely have enough to feed myself, and I only have one spoon."

I was being truthful. The can was small—seven ounces to be exact.

"One spoon. What's that supposed to mean? You don't want my fucking germs on your spoon? You too good to share your food with me?"

"Listen," I said as calmly as possible, "if I had more, I would share it, but this is all I have, and I'm not giving anything to anyone."

"That's cold-blooded. You got plenty in that can. You got to share with your people on the street. We're all family, bro."

I wondered if he was going to try to take the Spam from me. I didn't know what I would do in that event. I decided not to say anything else. I couldn't reason with him. Maybe I was being selfish, but I was hungry, and the can didn't hold much. I started eating faster, spooning it into my mouth. I had wanted to enjoy this meal casually, but I felt I needed to finish it as quickly as possible.

The guy got tired of waiting and gave me some unsolicited advice. "You're one selfish motherfucker. You'll get yours, man. Sooner or later, you'll be hungry, and nobody's gonna share their food with you. You can't be that way on the street. You need to make friends out here. You can't have no enemies."

I said nothing, and he finally walked off, disgruntled and hungry.

I was glad he was gone and I devoured the last few spoonfuls. I finished the can, threw it in the trash, and wiped the spoon clean. I kept it, just in case, and walked off to enjoy a couple more swigs. As the night wore on, I continued intermittently taking drinks. Just before midnight, I finished the last of the fifth. My booze was gone.

By 1:00 a.m., everyone had disappeared. I headed off, without a destination, pondering my bleak future. As I ventured south of Broadway, I heard someone calling to me. I turned around and spotted a young guy. He was clothed in a surprisingly clean, navy blue, hooded parka that was in remarkably good condition. He was wearing a large, sturdy backpack that looked pretty well stuffed.

"Hey, dude, what's up? Ya want some company? It's not too safe around here at night."

"Hey," I said. "Yeah, I guess you're right. Sure, I could use the company. It's pretty lonely out here."

He smiled. He was just a kid; maybe twenty, twenty-one. We were standing in an empty parking lot. I noticed that the building across the lot was the Prince Albert. I was near the hotel, looking at the rickety fire escape, and was pretty sure I could locate the window of my old room. A wave of something resembling nostalgia swept over me. Life at the Prince Albert was a nice alternative to the streets.

"Name's Eric," the kid said.

We shook hands.

"I'm Rob. Nice to find a friendly face."

"Yeah, I know what you mean, but you can't be too trusting. Lots of bad folks out here. How long you been on the streets?"

"This is my first night. I don't know how people can do this."

"Well, it beats the shelters, at least as far as I'm concerned."

"Does it?" I asked. "I was seriously considering checking one out. What don't you like about them?"

"Well, first off, they stink. Either B.O., disinfectant, or both. And most of the people are pretty sketchy. Always looking for an angle or with a favor to ask. But probably the number one reason that I avoid the shelters is that they don't let you in if you've been drinking, and I need to be drunk 24/7. My body needs the alcohol. No lie."

"Yeah, I know what you mean. I can't stop either. I don't know what I'll do now that my money's gone. I was staying right up there." I pointed toward a dark window.

Eric laughed. "The Prince Albert. Yeah, I've been there. Quite the palace. Is Frank still manning the desk?"

I smiled and nodded.

"Yeah, old Frank, he's quite a guy, isn't he?" Eric said.

"Yup, swell guy. I'll miss him."

I checked my watch; it was 1:45.

"Got somewhere to be?"

"No, I just like to keep track of time. No reason."

"Not to change the subject, but I've got a little something to keep us warm."

He unzipped his pack and pulled out a bottle.

I smiled. "T-bird," I said.

"Good old American bum wine. Screw-cap," Eric said. "Guaranteed to cure what ails you."

I chugged some and shuddered. It tasted like fruit-flavored kerosene. Still, I knew it would help me maintain my buzz. I passed it back to Eric.

"Some pretty harsh shit, but ya can't beat the price," he said. "Eighty cents a pop."

He gulped some down, grimaced, and puckered his lips.

"So, you wanna kill this shit or milk it?" he asked.

I laughed. "Let's kill it."

"Yeah, let's kill this bad bird."

He took a long draw and passed me the wine. It wasn't long before the T-Bird lay empty on the ground. This shit knocked me on my ass. I was extremely drunk and dizzy. I could see that Eric was enjoying the same effects. Despite my intoxicated state, I started to tremble from the cold.

"Dude, don't you have anything warm to wear?"

"No," I said, "I didn't think I would wind up on the street."

Once again, he reached into his backpack, and he presented me with a worn and soiled, salmon-colored Members Only jacket and a ratty gray sweatshirt. I accepted them gratefully and put on the jacket over the sweatshirt. I was still cold, but this was a big improvement over what I had been wearing.

"Wow, thanks, man. You don't know what a difference this makes. By the way, I really like your coat. I'm not asking for it or anything, but how'd you get it?'

"I showed up at the Sally at just the right time."

He was referring to the Salvation Army. That was the place to go for second-hand shoes, clothes, food, and, if you didn't mind the praying, a cot for the night. Eric had scored himself a very nice coat.

"Yeah, you oughta check it out. See if you can get something warm. The Goodwill runs thrift shops, too. I bought these boots there. Pretty nice, hunh?"

He was sporting what looked to be a brand-new pair of top-quality hiking boots.

"Very nice," I said.

"I love these boots. Only cost me ten bucks. They probably go for a hundred retail."

"If you don't mind my asking, how do you get the money to pay for stuff? You know, shoes, clothes, food, booze?"

"No, I don't mind, and I'm glad you asked. You've got to know where to go to survive in San Diego, especially in the winter. I go to churches and other places for sandwiches and soup. If you stay the night at the shelters, they give you supper and breakfast. But, like I said, I try to steer clear of them.

"My main source of income comes from selling plasma. There are a few places that pay for it. I like to use a clinic in El Cajon. It's nicer than the rest of them."

"What kind of money can you make selling plasma?"

"Well, they all pay about the same. Twenty-five bucks for the first time you donate. The first time's a hassle. They do a quick physical, blood test for AIDS and hepatitis, and they give you a piss test. It takes about two hours. After that, you can donate twice a week. They give you twelve bucks the first time and fifteen bucks the second time. So what's that, um, twenty-seven a week. If I'm careful, it pays for my alcohol and some food."

"But what if you've been drinking? Do they still let you donate?"

"If they smell booze on you, they won't let you donate, and you'll have to come another day with no booze on your breath. So I don't drink in the mornings when I sell my plasma. The place where I go opens at 7:00, so I get there early before I start coming down too hard. If you're shaky and your pulse is over 100, or if your blood pressure is way up, they won't take you either. Sucks when that happens, so I'm pretty careful about getting in and out early."

"Man, I don't know if I could stop drinking long enough to go through all the tests and shit. I get real shaky when I don't drink."

"Yeah, I feel for you, bro. I know how bad the jonesing can be. Another way to get some money is to panhandle, you know, fly a sign. 'Will work for food. God Bless.' You know, the stuff guys write on their cardboard. I don't like flying a sign, but when I'm desperate, I'll hit people up for spare change. Most people get scared off or hostile when you ask them for money. You gotta have a real thick skin, or be pretty lit, to panhandle."

"Yeah, I think I'd have to be pretty wasted to do that. If I'm crashing, there's no way I could do it."

"Yeah, alcoholism is hell. But, how to quit? I have no idea."

"I don't think I can."

He laughed. "Truth be told, I don't want to quit.

"So," he asked, "where do you plan on spending the rest of the night?"

I remembered that I had left the Prince Albert without turning in my key. With the high I had going, I bravely considered using it to spend the cold early morning in my old room. The key not only worked on my room door, but it also opened the door to the main entrance.

"Man, I should have thought of this earlier. I still have my key to the Prince Albert. I think I'll sneak upstairs for the night and duck out quick before it gets light. You're welcome to use the room if you want."

"You know what? That sounds cool. I haven't slept indoors in I don't know how long."

"Yeah, and it's cold as hell out here."

"Well, my man, what are we waiting for? Let's book us a room at the Prince Albert Hotel."

We both laughed. I trusted Eric. There was just something about him that put me at ease. We headed out of the parking lot and around the corner to the front entrance of the hotel.

"Ready?" I asked. I reached into my pocket and pulled out the hotel key.

"Yeah. Nobody's gonna be at the desk at two in the morning. Especially not Frank. Let's do it."

We climbed the cement steps to the front entrance. I slipped in the key and unlocked the door. We were in. I unlocked the next door, and we crept up the stairs to the second floor.

"Man, this is easy," Eric whispered.

"Yeah, c'mon. Let's go. My room's right here. Number 21."

"Shit," Eric said, "what if somebody is staying in your room?"

"Then I guess we'll have to get the hell out of here."

"Screw it," he said, "let's just do this. I'm drunk, and I'm tired."

I shoved in the key and opened the door. The room was dark. We hustled in, and I flipped on the light switch. Thank God, the room was empty. I quickly locked the door behind us.

He looked at the twin-size bed; no room for two. "Um. Bed's a little small," he said.

"You can have the bed," I said. "I'll sleep on the floor."

"No, man, that's okay. After all, it's your bed."

"Used to be. It's not mine anymore. You take the bed. You've already shared your wine and given me warm clothes. You deserve it."

"Tell you what," he said. "I'll take the floor, and I get the pillow. I'm used to sleeping on the ground, but I have to admit, a pillow sure would be nice."

"It's a deal," I said. "Take a blanket too."

"Okay. Sounds like a plan."

Eric sat on a chair and took off his boots and socks. He placed them under the old desk. He found a spot on the floor and lay down, wrapped in an old brown flannel blanket, his head resting comfortably on the pillow.

"Ahhh . . . man. It's been a while since I slept in such comfortable digs."

I checked my watch one last time. It was 2:15. I fell quickly to sleep. I'm pretty sure Eric did as well. I slept soundly. The T-Bird had done its job. I slept through the sunrise until I awoke to a rather loud conversation just outside my door. I wondered if Frank or one of the other desk clerks was aware that I was back, sleeping in my old room. I was anxious. I looked at my hands. They were trembling.

I wondered if Eric was awake too, and was surprised to see that he was not in the room. I thought that he might have gone to use the restroom. Maybe that was what the noise was about. Maybe he got caught sneaking around the second floor. But the room key was still on the nightstand, and the pillow and blanket he'd used were back on the bed. He'd even covered me with the blanket.

I looked at the time; 8:30. Jeez. I'd planned on waking up before seven. I sat upright on the bed, trying to hear the exchange outside my room. The talking had grown quieter, and the voices were more relaxed.

I checked the pockets of my jeans. The 75¢ was still there. I was relieved. I had enough to buy a 16-ounce can of beer. Not much, but better than nothing.

Then, to my amazement, I spied an unopened half-pint of vodka positioned securely on top of the desk. I sprang out of bed. Under the bottle was a scrap of brown paper with a message written on it. I picked up the note. It said:

"Good morning, Rob. Thought you could use an eye-opener. This ought to help. Enjoy your day and stay safe. Thanks for sharing your room. Peace."

Wow, this guy was something else. He knew what I was going through because, sadly, he was a fellow drunk. I wondered if I'd ever get the opportunity to thank him. In any event, I was sure he had Karma on his side. I hoped his situation would improve and that he would find his way off the streets. He was a young guy, and he still had a chance.

I wondered what time Eric had left. I guessed he didn't want to get caught by Frank, who probably would have broken his neck. I didn't even know if he used the door or the window. I figured if he left early enough, while it was still dark, he'd have gone out through the lobby. If he heard the same voices I did, he probably used the fire escape.

I went to the sink, splashed some water on my face, and sipped some from the faucet.

I needed an exit plan. No, I needed an escape plan. How the hell was I going to get out of there without being waylaid by Frank?

I looked out the window. The fire escape platform was right outside. But the stairs were barely attached to the wall, and I couldn't even spot a ladder. If I didn't want a broken leg, or worse, I'd have to use the door.

I decided to get dressed and ready before I opened my gift. I put on my pants, sweatshirt, and jacket. I grabbed the bottle with both hands and held it to my nose, inhaling its pungent bouquet. I sat on the bed, put the bottle to my lips, and guzzled it down. My throat burned raw, but I welcomed the sting.

I sat on the bed and waited for the warm cloak of composure to envelop me. Within minutes, I was feeling much better, and it was time to go. I approached the door. There was still some sort of discussion taking place, pretty loud, maybe angry. I could distinguish Frank's strong, bellicose voice. It was not what I wanted to hear.

I thought my pounding heart was going to burst. I took some slow, deep breaths, opened the door, and dashed to the staircase. I could see Frank off to the side. He immediately started yelling.

"Hey! You mother-fucking, low-life piece of shit . . ."

I was already running madly down the stairs, quickly out the door, and onto the sidewalk. I kept running until I was almost to Broadway, a few blocks away. I wondered if Frank would call the cops, or worse, try to find me himself. I dropped the key in a trash can and kept my pace to a good clip.

CHAPTER 19

Smithereens

Running out on the rent at the Prince Albert was a dangerous undertaking, but I had avoided the wrath of Frank. Once I had walked a few more blocks, I began to relax. I was still pretty drunk from guzzling the vodka, and I studied the throng of pedestrians, mostly professionals and office workers, walking to their jobs.

I considered the crowd as it came and went, and I tried to determine what type of person might be inclined to spare some change. I hadn't showered, shaved, or brushed my teeth, and the clothes that Eric had given me were ragged and dirty. There was a chill in the air. I estimated the temperature to be in the low fifties, and I was grateful for the extra clothing, dirty or not.

Eventually, a plain-looking young woman, wearing a brown cloth coat and sporting running shoes, approached. I moved slowly toward her, and when she met my gaze, I asked if she had any spare change so I could buy breakfast. She glared at me and walked away. I was humbled but not surprised. That was my first and last attempt at panhandling.

I sat on a bench at a city bus stop that had been "bum-proofed," which meant that there were metal armrests situated in a manner that prevented anyone from sleeping on it. Although San Diego had a very large homeless population, it was certainly not "homeless-friendly." I'd heard a rumor that the San Diego Police had a policy of rounding up homeless folk and sending them to Tucson with a one-way Greyhound ticket. This all reinforced my grim notion that I would not prevail on the streets. My go-to strategy was to find my brother Kevin and ask him for help. But I was *persona non grata* at the house in La Mesa. Moreover, the walk from downtown to their house was at least twelve or thirteen miles. But I had no choice; Kevin was my last chance.

I began walking from the bus stop on Broadway to Fifth Avenue, then east about two miles to Balboa Park. As I crossed the Cabrillo Bridge over the freeway, I was struck by the notion that the bridge was high enough for a jumper to commit suicide. I later learned that it was nicknamed "Suicide Bridge."

I headed north on Park Boulevard to the seamy University Park area. The vodka rush I had enjoyed earlier was fading. I looked for a liquor store and chose a rundown place whose sign read: "Beer. Wine. Liquor. Open at 6:00 A.M." I entered the dark little store and with my last 75¢, I purchased a 16-ounce can of Budweiser.

I left the store, ducked into an alley, popped the top, and guzzled the beer. I ditched the empty can and continued my journey to La Mesa. I remembered that the house in La Mesa was a few miles north of San Diego State University. I walked into a gas station and asked the clerk how far I was from the campus.

The clerk was a pleasant Black woman with a short, gray Afro. She looked at me and smiled. "Son," she said, "we are a good six miles from the University. Lucky for you, there's a bus that goes straight to the school from here."

I thanked her and left the store. I pretended that I was going to take the bus. I was embarrassed that I didn't have the fare. It was noon; I was on pace to reach SDSU around 2:00. Once I reached the University, I would have two and a half miles to go, which meant I'd reach the house just after 3:00, not exactly the best time to show up. I maintained an unhurried pace. I was in no rush to reach my destination.

Soon, I arrived on campus. I was reminded of my time at the University of Illinois. I watched the students, good-looking kids, each with somewhere to go, something important to do. In my dirty clothes, I felt like a leper. My alcohol high was completely gone. I was edgy, and I wanted to get away from there as quickly as possible. I did not belong there.

Just past 2:30, I was finally off-campus. I stayed on College Avenue, the most direct path to Lance Place, which was where Kevin, my father, and the others lived. I was dying for a drink. I reached their neighborhood and made my way to Princess Del Cerro Park. In better times, Kevin, Kerry, Kathy, and I used to play baseball there with my dad, Joanne, and her son. The park was only a few blocks from their home. It was almost 3:30, and the sun would be setting in about an hour. I figured the temperature to be about 50°. I could not show up until early the next morning when everyone was asleep, so I decided to spend the night at the park. I chose a pink concrete table to sleep on when the evening grew darker, and I wouldn't be seen.

When darkness fell, I slept fitfully, waking often. As it grew colder, I huddled into a ball but could not get warm. I checked my watch constantly, wondering if morning would ever come. The eastern sky gradually brightened, and I gazed at the glorious sunrise. By 6:30, there was a steady stream of warmly clothed joggers running laps around the park. I knew that my lying on the table would draw unwanted attention, so I rose, stretched my stiff muscles, and took a seat on a bench, trying to get warm. I was shivering like crazy. I knew it was time to see Kevin and ask for help, and I dreaded what lay ahead. Kevin would be sleepy and more than a bit cranky. But I knew what I had to do.

It was a short walk to Lance Place. I arrived at the house and detected no activity. I went to the side of the house and let myself into the backyard through a red cedar gate. Fortunately, Kevin's bedroom had a set of sliding glass doors that faced the yard. This meant I wouldn't have to meet him at the front or back door. I stepped onto the patio just outside his room. I knew that Kevin was not going to appreciate being awakened by his dirty, scruffy, homeless brother.

But I'd already come a long way and was out of options. I tapped on Kevin's window and waited. Nothing. I tapped a little harder, and a light went on. The curtain opened just a bit, and I recognized his girlfriend, Cheryl. She was barely awake, but she signaled for me to wait. I guessed correctly that she was going to wake Kevin. My stomach was in knots. I thought I was going to puke.

As I stood outside shaking, Kevin slid open the door. Cheryl had gone back to bed, and Kevin wasn't inviting me in.

"Rob, what are you doing here? You look terrible."

"I'm so sorry. I couldn't find a job, and I ran out of money. I got evicted from the Prince Albert."

"Damn, Rob. So, you're broke again? What are you gonna do now?"

"I don't know," I said.

"How did you even get here?"

"I walked."

"You walked from downtown? That's like fifteen miles. Where'd you spend the night?"

"At the park. On a picnic table."

"Wow." Kevin shivered. "It's gotta be like 30 degrees out here."

"I'm freezing," I said.

"Man, Dad's gonna shit if he sees you here."

"Yeah. I know I can't stick around."

"When's the last time you ate?"

"Umm . . . last night. I had a can of Spam."

"A can of Spam? Shit, Rob, did you spend all your money on booze? You can't keep doing this to yourself. Have you been drinking this morning?"

"No, I'm flat broke. I had some vodka yesterday morning and one can of beer about noon. I sure could use a drink."

He scowled. "Look, Rob, I'm not getting you any alcohol. You have got to stop drinking, get yourself together."

"I don't know if I can just stop drinking. I'm coming down real hard." I was telling the truth.

Kevin didn't understand the dynamics of alcohol withdrawal. "Well, you're just gonna have to tough it out. I can't keep contributing to your drinking problem. You can quit if you try hard enough. If you really want to stop."

I didn't say anything. I knew that his mind was made up, and I was in for an awful detox.

"Well, why don't you head back to the park and wait for me? I have to tell Cheryl what's going on," he said.

I asked, "Do you have any of my clothes? You know, jeans, sweatshirts, and stuff?"

"Yeah, I've got a few of your things in my closet. Dad and Joanne wanted to throw them in the trash, but I snagged them."

"Thanks, Kev, for everything. I hate to put you in the middle of this." I turned and left, heading back to the park.

"I'll get there as soon as I can," he called.

I made my way to the park and took a seat on a concrete bench that was soggy with dew. My pants were wet, and I was chilled to the bone. Kevin arrived half an hour later in his blue Mazda. He was a sharp dresser, with a pretty girlfriend and a well-paying job that he enjoyed. I wondered how my life had gone so wrong. He parked the car and walked toward me. He was carrying jeans, a jacket, and a sweatshirt.

"Rob, Rob, Rob . . . what are we gonna do with you?"

His mood was better. I was relieved.

"You should've just left me in Chicago," I said. "I know I'm a fucking pain in the ass."

"Aww, I love you, ya big lug." Kevin was the consummate salesman, always the schmoozer.

"I appreciate the kind words." God knows, I did. I felt like crying, just breaking down right there, and bawling like a baby.

"I gotta ask you," he said. "Where in the hell did you get that disgusting sweatshirt and jacket? And your jeans? They're filthy."

"Some guy gave them to me the other night. It was freezing, and I had nothing to wear but a T-shirt. He was a nice guy. A kid. I hope he's okay out there."

"Well, I brought you some fresh clothes. Do me a favor. Take off those rags and stuff them in the trash can."

I did as I was told. I took off the jeans and the dirty, crusty tops and put on a fresh pair of Levis along with a sweatshirt and a clean, warm winter coat.

"Okay, our number one priority is to get some food in that belly of yours. You're so skinny. That's quite a diet you've come up with. Maybe you should write a self-help weight-loss book."

"Yeah," I said. "We could call it 'Drink Yourself Thin.'"

"Bestselling title; can't lose. C'mon, Rob, let's get you some breakfast. How does an Egg McMuffin with some hash browns sound?"

"That would hit the spot," I said. But what I wanted, what I needed, was some vodka to soothe my writhing nerves. There was no way in hell that Kevin was going to buy me that. He was a great brother, and he had a huge heart, but he had no idea how badly my body needed alcohol.

We stopped at a McDonald's near the university and pulled into the drive-thru lane. Kevin ordered four Egg McMuffins, four orders of hash browns, and a large coffee with cream. "Do you want a coffee?" he asked.

"Oh, God, no. I think if I had any coffee, I'd jump right out of my skin. May I please have a Sprite?"

"Sprite it is."

We got our food and parked in the McDonald's lot. I wolfed down two McMuffins. The hash browns disappeared quickly as well.

"Wow. You were hungry."

"Famished," I said.

"Here," he said, "I can't eat my second McMuffin."

I took it from him gratefully.

When my stomach was full, Kevin said, "So we need to find you a place to stay. I'm kind of low on cash, so we have to think cheap. Let's see where we can get you an affordable room. Not downtown. We don't want to do that again. We can probably find a motel on Interstate 8 close to Jack Murphy Stadium."

I cringed at the thought of asking for a very big favor, but I knew I had to.

"Do you think we could stop at a liquor store? I'm coming down pretty hard, and a twelve-pack of beer would sure smooth me out."

Kevin didn't try to hide his irritation.

"We have got to get you off the sauce, Rob. I'm not going to buy you a twelve-pack of beer. No way I can do that."

"I'm gonna need something," I said. "Maybe a six-pack?"

"Look at yourself, Rob. You have to stop drinking. I'll buy you one quart of beer, that's all."

"Please, Kev, I'm gonna need more than a quart to detox myself."

"Listen, Rob, all I'm going to get you is a quart of beer. You'll just have to drink it slow, make it last. And you'll need lots of sleep. You can do this."

I resigned myself to the fact that I wasn't going to get more than a quart. Better than nothing, I told myself.

Kevin pulled into a 7-Eleven near the university. He went in and came out with a quart of Miller. My heart sank, but I thanked him. He thought he was doing the right thing. We got on the interstate and drove west. It wasn't long before we came upon a string of budget motels. We exited at Mission Gorge. Kevin pulled into the parking lot of a no-frills place and told me to stay in the car. He got out and walked to the office. Within minutes, he headed back to the car and handed me a key card. "You're in room 212," he said. "They're letting you check in early. It's almost 9:00; normal check-in is 3:00 p.m. I got you a room for three nights. That should give you enough time to get yourself together. You know, smooth out the shakes and all. Let's go find your room."

We got out of the car, and I was relieved that my room was on the top floor of the two-story motel. That meant I wouldn't be disturbed by any footsteps above me. I inserted my card, and we walked in. Considering how I had been living the last few weeks, this was a very nice arrangement. The carpet was clean, as was the comforter, and the TV had cable. I checked the bathroom. Everything looked freshly scrubbed. There were two drinking glasses wrapped in plastic and a new roll of toilet paper on the vanity.

"Not too bad, eh?" Kevin asked.

"No, this is great. Thanks, Kev."

"Well, I gotta go home and get ready for work. I'll stop by around 5:00 or so. I'll bring you dinner. Burger King okay?"

"Yeah, Burger King would be great."

"May I have your order, please?"

I laughed. "May I have a Whopper with cheese, small onion rings, and a regular Sprite?"

"You got it, sir. I'll see you in a few hours. Get some rest, watch a little TV. Just chill."

"Wait," I said.

"Yeah?" Kevin asked.

"I just want you to know how much I appreciate all that you're doing for me. Someday, somehow, I'm gonna make it up to you."

He hugged me. "Just get yourself better," he said.

I choked back my tears. God, how I loved him. Kevin left, and I was alone. I studied the quart of beer. I knew I was going to come down hard. I'd just have to make the best of it. I picked up the bottle, unscrewed the cap, and took a long pull. It tasted wonderful. I planned to take short sips, make it last a few hours. And that's what I somehow managed to do.

I expected some symptoms of delirium tremens within the next few days. DTs are a rough ride with the shakes and the hallucinations that come with them. Audio, visual, or tactile—they are extremely unpleasant, often nightmarish sensations.

Then, there was the possibility of a seizure. I knew that alcohol seizures usually occurred from around 24 to 72 hours after your last drink. They're known as tonic-clonic seizures. They used to be called grand mal seizures, but now they're tonic-clonic. I suffered one in 1984 on my third day without a drink. I was alone in my kitchen and was lucky to have suffered only a banged-up and bleeding head. I didn't need an ambulance.

I lay on the bed and tried to put thoughts of seizures and DTs out of my head. I finished the quart by 3:00. A quart of beer had never lasted me five hours. I dozed off with the TV on.

At 6:00, I was awakened by Kevin knocking on the door. He'd brought the food I'd asked for.

"So, how long did the beer last?"

"Amazingly, it lasted me five hours," I said.

"How are you feeling?"

"I've been better, but I didn't expect a cakewalk."

"I know you can do it. Just hang in there," he said. "Well, I can't stay. Cheryl's waiting in the car. I'll call you tomorrow morning, around 8:00."

"Okay, sounds good. Thanks, Kev, for everything."

"Just get some rest. I'll talk to you in the morning."

After Kevin left, I turned on the television. I clicked through all the channels, but I couldn't concentrate on anything. I turned off the TV and lay in bed trying to fall back to sleep.

The textured, white ceiling was undulating like the slow ripples of a small pond. I knew that it was my mind playing tricks on me, so I just focused on the waves and tried to enjoy the experience. If this was the onset of the DTs, it was starting gently.

At some point, I fell asleep. When I awoke, I was surprised to see that it was almost 2:00 a.m. I turned on the TV and was channel-surfing when I stopped on a station where a movie, *Smithereens*, was just beginning. The opening music was by the Feelies, an indie-punk band with a frenetic sound that complemented my jangled state of mind. The name of the song was tailor-made for me: "The Boy with the Perpetual Nervousness."

The movie was filmed in the early eighties and tells the story of a girl named Wren, who is trying to land a position as an agent or manager for a punk rock band. She has no experience and is turned down time and again throughout the movie. Wren meets a sweet young guy from Montana, who is living in his van in a parking lot frequented by prostitutes. The girls' pimp wants to buy the van.

The kid has a crush on Wren and lets her crash in his van. She is only using him, just like she uses everybody else. She sponges off her sister until the sister's husband puts an end to it. And her landlady evicts her for being far behind on the rent. The movie ends when the kid from Montana sells the van to the pimp and leaves New York to move back west. Wren finally has nowhere to go and no one left to use. She is homeless, alone, and vulnerable. Just deserts, I reckoned.

I was struck by the similarity between Wren's using everybody and my own bad behavior. I felt a connection to her. Like Wren, I was just getting by, sponging off of everybody, and always angling for a handout. The movie affected me and shamed me deeply.

Afterward, I watched a bunch of bad TV. None of it interested me, but I could not sleep. I lay awake throughout the night, wondering what just deserts lay ahead for me.

The next morning, Kevin arrived with two Egg McMuffins, hash browns, and a Sprite. I was feeling queasy, but I thanked him for his kindness.

"How about I bring a pizza after work, and we have dinner together?" he asked. "I'll get a Sprite for each of us. What do you want on it?"

"Pepperoni and mushrooms would be great," I said.

"Okay. I'll see you at six with a *deliziosa* pizza."

"Thanks, Kev. I hope you have a great day."

Once Kevin left, I unwrapped a McMuffin and took a small bite. I knew I had to eat to build up my strength. I finished the sandwich and two hash browns and put the second McMuffin on a counter. The Sprite was the best part of my breakfast. It helped settle my stomach. I placed the "Do Not Disturb" sign on my door handle, took a quick shower, and went back to bed. I didn't sleep much, but I knew that, in my situation, the passing of time was my ally.

I stayed in bed until 5:00, then dressed and watched the news. Kevin arrived at 6:00. He was carrying a large pizza and a two-liter bottle of Sprite. He grabbed the ice bucket, stepped outside, and returned to fill two glasses with ice and Sprite. As we ate slices of pizza out of the box, Kevin told me that he had some good news.

"So, Rob, get a load of this. Dad and Joanne found out that you'd been to the house, and they were fucking pissed. Kerry and Kathy took my side, and Dad told us we had until the beginning of January to move out. All three of us—and Cheryl. So, we're going to find a house around Kearny Mesa, maybe Clairemont Mesa. We're gonna get a place with four bedrooms so you can live with us. We'll keep you on the right track, help you look for work. I talked to Brian Rossi from work, and he said that you can stay with him and his girlfriend, Lisa, until we find a place. Brian's a great guy. They live in El Cajon, not all that far from the house. You wouldn't be there long, a couple of weeks. What do you think?"

"I don't know what to say, Kev. I think you're giving me a chance that I don't deserve, but after all you've done for me, all you're still doing, I'll do my best to stay off the sauce. Maybe even find some A.A. meetings."

"That's just what I wanted to hear," he said. "So you have tonight and tomorrow to get yourself together. I'll bring you breakfast and dinner tomorrow, and Friday morning I'll take you to El Cajon."

CHAPTER 20

Jim Beam and the Last Burned Bridge

After three nights in the motel, I was pretty much out of the woods as far as my alcohol detox was concerned. I moved in with Kevin's friend, Brian, and his girlfriend, Lisa, in El Cajon while Kevin, Kerry, and Kathy searched for a large house to rent.

The couple lived in a one-bedroom apartment, so I slept on their living room sofa. I took Eric's advice and found a place where I sold my plasma twice a week. I was paid twenty-seven dollars a week for "donating" each Monday and Thursday morning. I used the money to drink beer at a park that was close to Brian and Lisa's apartment.

In the middle of January, Kevin found a nice, five-bedroom house on Clairemont Drive just off Balboa Avenue. Brian and Lisa were invited to move into the new home. Altogether, the house was occupied by Kevin, Cheryl, Kerry, Kathy, Brian, Lisa, and me. I found a warehouse job just north of Clairemont Mesa Boulevard and rode a ten-speed bike to work each day. And, each day after work, I would visit a liquor store to buy a six-pack of beer and a half-pint of vodka, which I would drink in a deserted field nearby. And each morning, I would wake up for work a nervous wreck.

Finally, one day, I awoke with such a bad case of the shakes that I could not go to work. I continued drinking and never returned to that job except to pick up my final paycheck. I was drunk when I showed up for the check.

The job market was pretty healthy in San Diego during the first months of 1987. I boozed my way through a string of warehouse and factory jobs and lost each one when I was too drunk or shaky to show up. I had some money put away, which I spent on booze. It was the only thing that mattered. Finally, by the end of April, I did nothing but isolate myself in my bedroom and drink cheap beer and vodka. Nobody knew what to do about me and my drinking.

One morning—it was a Monday, May 4—I awoke at 5:30 in a cold sweat. I had felt something run across my chest, and it was scurrying on my bedroom floor, ducking underneath my bed. I sat up, but could no longer see what I was pretty sure was a gecko-sized lizard, or maybe a chameleon.

I crouched on the floor, hoping I wouldn't find anything. I had heard scratching sounds inside the walls throughout the night and early morning, but this was the first time that I had seen something. I hadn't had a drink in about seven hours and realized I might have been imagining the sounds emanating from the wall as well as my sighting of the reptile. I wanted to crawl back into bed, fall asleep, and forget that unpleasant incident.

But I was out of alcohol. I had nothing to soothe my writhing nerves, not even a single beer. I could not return to sleep. So, I sat up in bed, scanning the room—floor, walls, and ceiling—hoping not to spot that fucking lizard.

I knew that the mini-mart a couple of blocks away would not be selling alcohol until six, so I'd have to suffer a bit longer. I nervously slid out of bed and made my way as quietly as possible toward the kitchen. Thankfully, everyone was still asleep. But Kevin always woke for work at 6:30. I had much to do in a very short time.

I gingerly opened the refrigerator door in search of beer. There wasn't a single bottle or can inside. I closed the fridge and scanned the living room for any partially filled bottles. There were two on the coffee table, both about one-third full and with cigarette butts floating in them. I was desperate, so I drank the first beer slowly until I snared two disgusting butts that I clenched between my teeth. I spit out the butts and guzzled the remaining beer. I repeated those steps with the second bottle.

This revolting effort had earned me about eight ounces of beer. I quickly and quietly returned to my room. Still scanning for the lizard, I put on a pair of dirty jeans and a T-shirt that hadn't seen the inside of a washing machine in several weeks. I rifled through my pants pockets and found a ten, two singles, and some change. I had more than enough to buy a twelve-pack of cheap iced beer, which at 5.5% alcohol delivered more bang for a buck than most beers. What it lacked in taste, it made up for in alcohol.

The morning sun hadn't risen yet, but the sky was growing lighter. As quietly as possible, I unlocked and slid open the glass door that faced the backyard. I decided it was best to leave it open. I knew I would be right back, and perhaps this would provide an exit for my creepy, green guest.

Next, I gently unbolted the wooden gate on the side of the house, leaving this open as well. I hurried, turned the corner, and walked to the gas station down the street. It was 5:55. *Fuck,* I thought, *they won't open the cooler for five more minutes.* That was an eternity, and I was feeling no relief from the rancid beer I had just consumed.

Finally, 6:00 arrived, and I entered the small store. The place was packed with people paying for coffee and gas. I made my way to the beer cooler, but it was still locked. Shit. I had wanted to make this purchase quickly and rush back home. I sheepishly asked an employee to open the cooler. He gave me a look that said, *"A little early for a beer, isn't it?"* I got that look a lot, and I never got used to it.

I followed him to the cooler, grabbed a twelve-pack, and waited nervously in line to make my purchase. Finally, I reached the register. The beer cost $9.76. With my shaking hands, I gave the clerk the wrinkled ten-dollar bill.

I grabbed the twelve-pack and the change and thanked him. As I made my way out, I felt that every coffee-drinking customer saw me for the alcoholic piece of shit I was. And, who was I to disagree?

Finally, I made it home, passed through the wooden gate, and slipped into my bedroom. I slowly closed the large, glass door, sat at the foot of my bed, and polished off three ice-cold beers. It took less than ten minutes to down them. I undressed and stashed the remaining beers under the bed. As a warm sense of relief coursed through my brain, I could hear a door open and close. It was Kevin getting up for work. I got into bed and pulled the blankets over my head.

My door opened, and while I pretended to be asleep, Kevin softly asked, "Is everything all right, Rob?"

I rubbed my eyes as if he had just awakened me.

"Oh, hi, Kev. Yeah, sure, everything's okay."

"Good. Get some rest and don't drink. I know it's tough, but you need to stay sober."

"I will," I lied.

"Good. Take care, buddy. Remember, I love you."

Kevin was so kind. I knew I was a loser alcoholic and that

I didn't deserve his kindness, but he didn't see me that way. Nevertheless, as soon as the door closed, I was on the floor pulling out another beer.

Despite all the kindness that Kevin continued to show me, I maintained my selfish ways. Kevin had been collecting Jim Beam decanters for some time, and he probably had twenty or so in his collection. They likely ranged in value from thirty to possibly several hundred dollars apiece. I didn't know the individual values of any specific decanters, but I knew that they were expensive collectibles. I guessed that their total value was at least $1500, maybe more. Kevin believed that the decanters were worthless if the seals were broken and the whiskey was gone. I would later learn that these collector items were supposed to be empty because they were made of china, and the whiskey would corrode them. Also, the whiskey caused the corks to dry out. But, at the time I was drinking all this whiskey, I was under the impression that my drinking was rendering the decanters worthless. I was a selfish jerk who was more concerned with staying drunk no matter the cost to my brother, who had helped me out of so many jams.

Each time I'd down the contents of a decanter, I would fill it with water and carefully twist the labels so that the tax seals appeared unbroken. However, after I had finished drinking the last of the collection, Kevin noticed one decanter where I had been sloppy, and the seal did not line up properly. He was furious, and he was at the end of his rope. The next day, Kerry and his girlfriend drove me to a detox center south of downtown. This would be the beginning of a very scary experience for me, a drunk who'd finally burned the last of his bridges.

CHAPTER 21

13th and Island Detox

The detox center was at the intersection of 13th and Island, right next to the trolley tracks. This was a squalid part of San Diego, but I was an equally squalid individual. Sam, a short, powerfully built man, about 60 years old, signed the necessary admission forms.

"Okay, do you go by Robert, Bob, or what?"

"Rob," I said.

"Okay, Rob. This place is pretty unique. Some people come here voluntarily for a three-day detox. Like you. If you're lucky, you get one of the rooms. Each has four beds, but there are only six rooms. If all the beds are full, you grab a mat, spray it down with Lysol, and find a place to sleep on your left side of this long red line. That line of red tape is all that separates you from the majority of our 'guests.' Ya see, this place also serves as a four-hour drunk tank for those blockheads the cops think aren't dangerous enough to lock up. If they get too rowdy, we call the cops, and they go to jail. So, for the most part, they're pretty obnoxious and rude, but only a handful a night actually wind up in a cell."

Only a handful. I shuddered.

"Ya know, this being Memorial Day Weekend and all, it's gonna be pretty crazy in here. The good news is that we have a room with an empty bed. It's yours for three nights. The noise from the trolley can be pretty annoying, but being in a room beats the hell out of sleeping in the common area. Believe me. You're gonna be comin' down pretty hard, aren't you? You ever get the DTs, seizures?"

"Both, mostly DTs."

"Rob, I wish we could give you something, but this goddamned place is strictly non-medical. We can't even give you Benadryl to help you sleep. Just try to stay calm and steer clear of the trouble-makers. We'll get you through this in one piece, trust me."

"Thanks, Sam. I really appreciate it," I said.

* * *

It was about noon. I'd made it through this drunk tank/detox Sunday and Monday nights, and Tuesday morning. I was still shaking like a motherfucker. A grubby-looking guy, about 50, sporting a week's worth of stubble and dirty gray hair, asked me if I wanted to play spades.

"Sure," I said. "But I'm pretty rusty. And shaky. I'm coming down pretty hard."

"Booze," he said, somewhat sympathetically. I nodded.

"Well, don't worry about it. We're all a bunch of hardcore drunks. My name's Ted. We're playing over at that table."

He motioned to a row of long, beat-up, dark brown Formica lunch tables, each of which seated about eight. The chairs were standard-issue, beige steel card-table variety. There were two pretty crusty-looking guys already seated at the table. They both needed a bath.

Ted and I sat on opposite sides of the table.

"Okay, me and uhh . . ."

"Rob," I said.

"Yeah, me and Rob will play you two guys. I forgot your names."

"Michael," said one.

"Bill," said the other. It was hard to believe, but he was shaking harder than I was.

Ted said, "Okay, we'll play to 500. I got the pencil and paper, so I'll keep score."

We were fine with that. He was the only one whose hands were steady enough to write anyway. We were one sorry foursome.

Ted shuffled and slid the deck for Bill to cut. Ted restacked it and dealt each of us thirteen cards; we weren't using jokers. As we gathered our cards, Bill's eyes rolled backward. All you could see were the whites. He made a kind of gurgling sound, which was barely audible among all the hubbub going on at the detox center. He fell straight back in his chair and smashed his head on the filthy linoleum-covered floor. He was bleeding pretty badly.

"He's having a seizure," I said. "He needs an ambulance."

Two staff members noticed the commotion and hustled to where Bill lay on the floor. Al, a short, fat guy, asked what had happened.

"I'm pretty sure he's having a seizure," I repeated. I was in a near panic.

"Yeah, must have had a pretty bad hand," Ted said. No one laughed.

Within minutes, fire department paramedics arrived, and after taking his vitals, they put him on a stretcher and left for the hospital. These same paramedics would be called back within an hour when a feeble old bum had what must have been a heart attack in the men's shower. He was dead when they wheeled him out.

CHAPTER 22

Serenity Springs

After spending three days safely ensconced in a four-bed room at 13th and Island, I was offered a spot at a small rehab next door called the Sobriety House. I would be there from Monday, June 1, until Monday, June 8. That meant that I would be allowed to stay at the detox center for five more nights. The problem was, I had used up my three days in a bedroom and would have to spend the next five nights on a mat on the floor, separated from the pandemonium of the drunk tank by the simple red line of tape. Those five days were no picnic, but they passed without calamity.

The Sobriety House was a calm refuge compared to the commotion and chaos at the detox center. The Sobriety House was clean, the food was good, and each bedroom only had two occupants. We watched educational films about alcoholism and addiction, and we had groups where we would discuss how to live sober once we were released.

On my third day at the Sobriety House, I was informed that there was an opening at a long-term men's rehab on a large tract of land about sixty miles east of San Diego. It was called Serenity Springs, and the average stay ran from three to four months. I had nowhere else to go, so I applied for a spot at the ranch, which housed about fifty men.

On Monday morning, the 8th, a large white van arrived to fetch me and another resident. The driver, Pete, was an upbeat guy who also served as the ranch custodian. He had been sober for almost two years and was a client at the Springs before he was hired on as a staff member. The concept of going two years without a drink was beyond my comprehension.

We were assigned rooms, and mine had four beds. To save space, we slept in bunk beds. The other three beds were already occupied, so I got a bottom bunk. I never felt comfortable with the guys I shared the room with, so I was only in there to sleep and dress.

The Springs hosted four mandatory Alcoholics Anonymous meetings each week—Sundays, Mondays, Wednesdays, and Fridays. Each meeting began at 7:00 p.m. and lasted an hour. The meetings were open to the public, but we didn't get many outsiders. The few we got were usually guest speakers or long-time A.A. members whose calling was "to carry the message to the alcoholic who still suffers." These folks were doing what they called service work, and they were moved to "share their experience, strength, and hope" with the motley crew that called Serenity Springs home. The meeting room, which also served as our cafeteria, could hold about 100 people.

We rarely saw any women, except for Betty, who was in charge of the Springs. Betty was a tough old gal, who, despite being only five feet tall and tipping the scales at about 90 pounds, could scare the bejeezus out of any man at Serenity Springs. She was intense and wore a constant frown. I adhered to all the rules and regularly volunteered to help when something needed doing, so I was pretty sure that I was on Betty's good side. And that was a good thing. She had a fierce temper and didn't hesitate to holler and cuss at anyone who pissed her off.

At the beginning of every A.A. meeting, someone would be asked to read the preamble, which took about five minutes to recite. I lived in morbid fear of reading that preamble. It reminded me of my first days of law school before I learned about the benefits of alcohol. My voice would crack and my hands would tremble like crazy whenever I was chosen to read it. So, I avoided this task like the plague.

I managed to make friends with the three guys whom I felt most comfortable with. Their names were Sebastian, Zach, and Ethan. All three were in their early twenties; I was thirty-one, but we got along well despite our age difference. There was an exercise area near the main house that was shielded from the harsh rays of the desert sun by a thick canvas tarp. We had a weight bench, barbells, and an assortment of dumbbells. We worked out there each afternoon around three o'clock, after our daily chores. And we finished exercising just before the dinner bell rang at five.

Sebastian was the youngest member of our group. He was a tall, thin, and extremely good-looking kid who had just turned twenty-one. Sebastian had been a heavy user of "speedballs," a liquid mixture of cocaine and heroin that is injected into a vein. From what I understood, speedballs packed a mighty strong punch. Sebastian took to forging checks to support his habit, and he was eventually arrested and sent to the Springs by a judge.

Zach was two years older than Sebastian. He had shoulder-length, sun-bleached hair, and he always wore tank tops to display his muscular arms and shoulders. He was pretty full of himself, but he wasn't a bad guy. I might have acted the same way if I were as handsome as he was. Zach was addicted to crack, which is cocaine that has undergone a process that allows it to be smoked rather than snorted. Smoking crack sends the drug to your brain in as little as eight seconds. When cocaine is snorted, it takes up to ten minutes. The downside of smoking crack is that its effect only lasts a few minutes. That's why addicts are constantly "chasing" their first high.

I felt closest to Ethan. He was twenty-five years old and was also a nice-looking guy. Pot and alcohol were his drugs of choice, and he had spent a lot of time in and out of hospitals and detox centers. Ethan was tall and thin and had beautiful gray eyes with long, thick lashes. He also had a very mellow disposition. I liked Ethan, and everyone else did too.

By far, my favorite thing about living at the Springs was the star-filled night sky, which was completely unspoiled by city lights. San Diego felt so far away, and the stars shone like sparkling diamonds spilled on a black velvet mantle. I spent many hours lying on my back and marveling at the beauty of our magnificent night sky.

Sebastian, Zach, Ethan, and I spent most of our evenings playing spades under those glorious stars. Occasionally, another client or two would drop by to shoot the breeze. My favorite encounter occurred one night when Clint, a strapping young guy from Nebraska, visited us. Clint grew up on an alfalfa farm, raising and preparing hay for horses, cattle, sheep, and goats. He would effortlessly load bales of hay weighing 70 to 80 pounds onto wagons that were pulled by huge tractors. Clint had competed in various bale tossing contests, and we were not surprised to learn that he had won many. He was a very strong young man.

One night, Clint regaled Sebastian, Zach, Ethan, and me with his hilarious account of a Sunday morning in a small Nebraska town when he woke up in a churchyard to the confused voices of a handful of kids who had discovered him. He awoke—better yet, he came to—squinting at the blinding morning sun. He stared at his watch, which read 8:45. As his eyes adjusted to the light, he saw that he was surrounded by a group of about thirty people—men, women, and children, all dressed in their Sunday best. To his absolute horror, he realized that he was buck naked, wearing nothing but his wristwatch. He thought he couldn't be more ashamed.

Then, he saw it. Next to one of his beat-up Nikes lay a steaming pile of shit, apparently some of his handiwork from the night before. Everything was a blur. How did he wind up at this church? Why was he stripped naked? And why, oh why hadn't he shown the good sense, even in one of his deepest stupors, to find some bushes where he could have taken a shit? But there he was in this pristinely kept, peaceful churchyard, without a stitch of clothing, while several dumbfounded, God-fearing Christians looked on.

"Do you think he's dead?" asked a little boy no older than six or seven.

"He's not dead. He's dead drunk," said a gruff old man. "We need to call the cops. Let's get the kids away from this disgusting piece of filth."

"'Disgusting piece of filth.' That's what they called me, and that's how I felt," Clint said.

It didn't take long for a squad car to arrive. Neither of the two young cops wanted to get close to him, and who could blame them? Noticing the festering heap of excrement and the absence of any toilet paper, or even leaves, they eyed each other, and one cop said, "Let's radio for an ambulance. Let 'em earn their paychecks."

"Yeah," added the second cop, "he's probably gonna need to detox anyway."

When the paramedics arrived, they were not pleased. "You assholes," groused a fireman. "You could have put him in your back seat."

"Look," said one of the cops, "you know he's gonna need detox. Besides, your stretchers are a lot easier to clean than our back seat."

"You're a dick," said the fireman.

"C'mon, now. Watch your language. We're at church," admonished the smiling cop.

We laughed so hard at Clint's deadpan depiction of that Sunday morning in the churchyard that we were in tears. Clint was a good sport and didn't mind our laughter. I'll never forget his sidesplitting story.

I stayed at the Springs from the eighth of June until August 31, when I was offered a position in San Diego as a live-in custodian at an A.A. Alano Club in Pacific Beach, just a two-block walk to the ocean. I jumped at the opportunity and was thrilled to learn that among the new custodians was Jim Sanders. Jim had been an aerospace engineer for several years until his drinking cost him his job, and he wound up driving a taxi. He was very bright and had a terrific sense of humor. Jim was in his mid-sixties, and, like Ethan, he was well-liked by everyone at Serenity Springs.

So, Jim and I moved to the Pacific Beach Alano Club. I was going to miss the friends I'd made at Serenity Springs. I would miss Ethan most of all. He promised to drop in on Jim and me, but he never did. I never saw any of the guys from Serenity Springs again. I hoped they would all do well, but, like at other rehabs, the success rate for guys who completed the program at Serenity Springs was not encouraging.

Jim and I worked hard at the Alano Club, and life was good. The club was very nice. On the first floor was an area with sofas and easy chairs, along with a large-screen television. The top floor had a meeting hall that could seat well over a hundred people. There was a small area where we prepared two large, commercial-sized coffee makers. We would make the coffee before each meeting and clean up when the meetings ended.

The room where we kept the coffee and supplies also held

dollies for storing and moving several large card tables and about 150 card table chairs. Before every meeting, we would roll the carts and the large tables out to the meeting room. And after the meetings, we would stack the chairs, wipe down the tables, and roll everything back to the storeroom.

The living quarters for the custodians were on the same floor as the meeting hall. We each had a twin bed and a dresser, and we shared a large closet that provided ample space. Back then, I didn't own many clothes, but we did have uniforms, which were sent out weekly to be dry-cleaned. The area was quite spacious, and the one bathroom we shared was large, with a two-sink vanity, a toilet, and a shower. We kept the bathroom spic and span.

Jim and I were very dependable, and we enjoyed our lives at the Alano Club, but we could never keep a regular third custodian. Guys would stay for a few weeks, then invariably fall back to drinking and using. Jim and I would often work extra shifts to make up for the regular absence of our third co-worker. But we didn't mind; we were good friends and we worked well together.

Jim was an outgoing guy; he could strike up a conversation with anyone. I, on the other hand, was painfully shy and a bundle of nerves. Jim loved to visit the high-priced art galleries in nearby La Jolla. I would join him fairly often, although I never felt comfortable in those tony shops. I felt like a fraud because I knew that I could never come close to paying for any of the art we viewed. I was that way no matter where I went. Whether I was at a clothing store or an auto dealership, I always felt an obligation to buy what was being sold.

On the first floor of the club, there was a very nice little Mexican restaurant that had eight tables, each of which sat four. The restaurant was owned and run by a terrific guy named Sergio. Jim and I bused tables, and each night we would sweep and mop the floors and make sure all the tables were cleaned. Sergio was very happy with our work, and he allowed us access to the kitchen to make ourselves snacks when we worked the overnight shift. We changed shifts every week so that no one would constantly be saddled with the overnight shift, which was, by far, the toughest.

Sergio was a great cook, and we received three free meals each day, seven days a week. He had two very nice waitresses working for him, Elena and Isabel. I liked Elena, who was almost like a mother to me. She could sense what a nervous guy I was, and she kept me on an even keel. I still look back on those days fondly, and I miss Sergio, Elena, and Isabel. Especially Elena.

In addition to the great food and free rent, we were paid $150 a week. This helped us save enough money for the day when our six-month tenure drew to a close, and we would have to find new places to live. Saving money was easy while working at the club. Jim and I both felt fortunate to be living and working there.

When February 1988 arrived, it was time to move on. I had decided to return to Chicago. Jim was going to stay with his son for a bit until he got back on his feet. During my last days at the club, I said farewell to all the friends I had made and the acquaintances I had met.

On Sunday, February 28, I said goodbye to Jim. I was going to miss him terribly, and I worried about his health and his sobriety. He was one of the best friends I'd ever had. Unfortunately, as it turned out, I would never hear from him again, and since I didn't have his son's address, I couldn't write him. And I never saw or heard from Elena, Sergio, Isabel, or anyone else I met at either Serenity Springs or the Alano Club. Having these great people absent from my life was the worst thing about leaving San Diego.

CHAPTER 23

Chicago Didn't Change, and Neither Did I

On February 28, my plane landed in Chicago, and my brother, Kurt, picked me up at the airport. He had a studio apartment in Forest Park that he never used since he had moved in with his girlfriend, Jane. He offered to let me live there rent-free while I looked for a job. But, Kurt insisted, I had to stay sober.

I soon found a job as an inventory clerk at a small screw and bolt packaging company in the nearby industrial suburb of Stone Park. The bus stop was only a few blocks from the apartment, and the bus ride to work was about half an hour long. Since I didn't own a car, this arrangement worked perfectly for me.

The company, Advantage Fasteners, was much smaller than Select. While Select had employed about 150 people, Advantage only had about twenty employees. Also, Select had entered the computer age in the early '80s, but Advantage still kept all its records on paper and Rolodex cards. It was an old-fashioned business, but everyone was very friendly, and I enjoyed the work.

There was a popular bowling alley across the street from my apartment building. I managed to maintain my sobriety and kept the job at Advantage until the middle of October, when I gave in to my cravings and crossed the street to enjoy a few beers. Forest Park had a lot of bars, and in the next few weeks, I visited many of them.

Unfortunately, I began waking up with the shakes and soon quit my job at Advantage. I spent all of my money on beer and vodka until one terrible morning when I was jonesing so badly that I decided to sell a silver coin that a diver friend had given me three years earlier. The coin was a piece of eight, for eight reales, and it weighed nearly an ounce. It had been recovered in 1985 from the remains of the wreck of the Spanish galleon, Nuestra Señora de Atocha (Our Lady of Atocha), which was the most widely known vessel of a fleet of Spanish ships that sank in a hurricane off the Florida Keys in 1622. The coin was in very good condition. I never knew its exact value, but it might have fetched from a few hundred to over a thousand dollars.

I had no alcohol or money, and I was suffering badly. I rifled through the Yellow Pages, looking for the nearest coin shop. I found one just a couple of blocks away. The man behind the counter recognized how bad off I was. He offered me a paltry twenty dollars for the coin, but I was hurting so badly that I said yes to his offer. I knew I'd been ripped off big time, but I was in no condition to do anything about it.

The booze I purchased lasted me two days. When I was again out of alcohol and money, I called Kurt, and he told me that I could move in with him, Jane, and Jane's young daughter, Stacy—provided, of course, that I lay off the alcohol. I had no choice but to accept Kurt's terms, and on Thursday, November 10, I moved out of the studio and into a converted bedroom in the attic of their Oak Park home.

I suffered through the next few days without a drink. I did not eat for over 72 hours. By Monday, the 14th, I felt that I'd weathered the worst of my alcohol detoxification, and I emerged from the attic to shower, shave, and brush my teeth. The following Sunday, I checked the Chicago Tribune classifieds for a job and found a warehouse position at a company called Danse, which made ballet slippers and accessories.

I took the bus to Danse early Monday morning and was hired to start the next day, November 22, two days before Thanksgiving. It was a small business, and I worked in the shipping and receiving department. I was friendly with two female co-workers. Paula was rather plain but very sweet. Emily was pretty and high-spirited, and she possessed an exquisitely droll sense of humor. She reminded me of Rosemary from Select Screw and Bolt. I had a crush on her, and I think that she might have had feelings for me.

Working alongside Emily was one of the things that helped keep me sober. One Friday morning, January 27, I asked Emily if I could borrow a dollar to buy a soda. She reached into her pocket and handed me a dollar bill.

"You'll be here bright and early Monday?" she asked. "You're not gonna run out on me?"

I laughed. I had no plans to miss work on Monday morning. But after my shift, I stopped at a bar next to the currency exchange where I cashed my paycheck. I got drunk and wound up spending three days at the Blue River Motel in Melrose Park. When I was a teenager, my friends used to throw New Year's Eve parties there.

I had taken a cab to the motel and stopped at a liquor store before arriving. I bought two 1.75 liters of vodka and a couple of two-liter bottles of 7 Up. The motel seemed to have fallen on hard times, as was evidenced by the nearly empty parking lot. When I checked in, my bags of booze and soda did not raise any eyebrows. I was a paying customer, and that was good enough.

I stayed drunk the entire weekend, but by Monday morning, I was broke and out of booze, so I checked out of the motel and trekked five miles through the ice and snow until I arrived at Kurt's house. When I showed up, Kurt was more relieved that I was safe than he was upset with me. Within a couple of days, he arranged for me to enter a 28-day rehab in the northwest suburb of Schaumburg. The place was called ACHIEVE. I was headed to rehab again.

CHAPTER 24

ACHIEVE

On an uncharacteristically mild Wednesday afternoon, February 1, 1989—the weather had reached the mid-sixties—Kurt delivered me to the admitting area at ACHIEVE. It was just before 4:00. I was toting a brown paper bag that contained two pairs of jeans, three sweatshirts, and some socks and underwear.

Kurt introduced himself to a staff member. "Hi, I'm Kurt Rickelman. I talked with Marsha about getting my brother a bed in your detox."

A woman said hello to Kurt. "Yes, she left a note. I'm Grace. And I assume that you're Robert." She was talking to me.

In a shaky voice, I said, "Yes, I'm Robert."

"Well," Grace said, "this is a 28-day detox and rehab. The total price for 28 days is $450."

"Four-fifty," Kurt said. "Do you accept personal checks?"

"Yes, we do," she said. "A personal check will be just fine."

Kurt handed her the check. "Do you need me for anything else?" he asked.

"No, we'll take it from here. Thank you for bringing Robert. We'll take good care of him."

"Thanks." Kurt turned to me. "So long, Rob. They're going to help you get yourself together." He hugged me, and I choked back my tears.

"Thanks for everything, Kurt. I love you. I'll pay you when I get out of here," I said. After working at Danse for three months and paying Kurt and Jane seventy-five dollars a week for room and board, I'd managed to put away nearly $900. I was eager to pay him what I owed.

"I love you, too. Get yourself better." He turned and walked away.

"Well, Robert, could I have your bag, please? We need to make sure you didn't pack any prohibited items," Grace said. I gave her the bag. She emptied everything, found no contraband, and put it all back.

"Russell, here, is our health aide. He's going to take your vitals."

I looked at Russell. He was huge—I mean, grossly overweight. I figured he weighed more than four hundred pounds. His shirt and jeans were filthy and stained. His hair was greasy, and he looked like he hadn't showered in days.

"Okay, Robert," Russell said, "take a seat here, and I'm going to check your vitals and give you a blood-alcohol breath test. I'm sure you've been told that we only accept patients who are completely sober. Why don't we do the breathalyzer first?"

He handed me a black instrument with a nozzle sticking out of one side.

"Just blow into the nozzle until I say stop."

I held the breathalyzer and blew into it for about five seconds until Russell said stop. He took the device from me and checked the LED readout. "Good news," he said. "You blew a zero. Looks like you are going to be our guest for the next four weeks."

I was relieved. I had been drinking so heavily recently that I wasn't certain that all the alcohol was out of my system.

"We need to get your vitals," Russell said. "First, we'll take your temperature." He placed a thermometer in my ear; it beeped, and he read it. "One hundred point one," he said, "you have a slight fever, which is typical for the first day of detox."

He wrapped a blood pressure cuff around my bicep and pumped a bulb. Soon after he released the pressure, he got his reading. "Holy cow! One ninety-five over one fifteen. We're going to have to keep an eye on you. And your pulse is 120, which is way too high. We'll be taking your vitals every two hours until they improve. That's it for now."

"Grab your things, Robert," Grace said. "I'll show you to your room."

I hesitated, then took a breath and asked, "Is this a medical detox? I mean, am I going to get something to calm my nerves? I'm shaking like a leaf."

"I noticed the shaking, but I hate to tell you that this is a non-medical detox. We don't have a license to give out medicine like sedatives or sleep aids. The first few days will be a rough ride. I'm sorry."

"But what if I have a seizure? I'm worried about having a seizure. I've been drinking heavily for a long time."

"Well, every once in a while, someone does have a seizure, and we call an ambulance. We have measures in place."

"What if I have one while I'm alone? Like in my room."

"You're worrying too much. Let's go find your room."

She led the way as we walked down a hallway of faded green walls and a dark brown and tan linoleum floor. I imagined that the building had once been a school, and old classrooms now served as clients' bedrooms. For some reason, that depressed me.

We stopped at room 10 and went inside. There were three beds. She pointed to one located against the farthest wall. "That will be yours for the next 28 days, Robert. Not luxurious, but better than being homeless."

"Yeah," I said. "Been there, done that."

"Well," she said, "you have lots of time to get yourself together, and we're going to do everything we can to get you clean and keep you clean. Okay, so why don't you put your things on your bed for now? It's just about dinner time. I'll show you to the cafeteria."

We walked on and reached the cafeteria. It had probably once been the school gymnasium. There was a long line of about twenty or so people. I took my place at the end.

"Enjoy your dinner, then get some rest," Grace said. And she left.

When I finally got to the head of the line, a middle-aged man wearing a hairnet and whose hands shook furiously, gave me a tray with a plate of corned beef hash and two cornbread biscuits. The place was full, so I took a seat at a table where three other patients were eating.

"Hey, you're new, huh? You can get a glass of juice over there," said a clean-cut guy who looked to be about my age. I got a glass and filled it at a dispenser situated on a long lunch table.

"Welcome to ACHIEVE. I'm Paul, this is Gary, and this is Lucy." The sight of Lucy was unsettling. Her entire face was horribly burned. She did not have a nose, and her right ear was missing. She also had no eyelids or eyebrows, and she was missing three fingers on her right hand and the thumb and index finger of her left. I tried not to stare as I was introduced to her. I shook Paul and Gary's hands and gingerly grasped what was left of Lucy's right hand. Then I turned to eat my supper. My hands were shaking like crazy.

"It really sucks that they don't give you anything for the shakes," Paul said. "I was in your shoes three days ago."

"Same here," Gary said. "They shouldn't make us go through

this without meds."

"Yeah," I said, "I could use something to help with these shakes."

"Just try to hang in there," said Lucy. She sounded sweet. I tried to concentrate on my food tray, but Lucy sensed that I was uncomfortable with her appearance.

"Well," she said, "I know it's hard not to wonder why I look like I do. So I'm going to come straight out and tell you."

She was right; I wanted to know what horrible thing had happened to her.

She began her story. "Three years ago, my husband announced that he was leaving me for another woman. I was devastated. The night he told me, I drove to a bar and got extremely drunk. When I left the bar, I got on the expressway and was speeding in my 1979 Volkswagen Beetle, a two-door convertible. I had my foot pressed on the gas. As I was approaching a large overpass, I knew what to do. With the car travelling at top speed, I aimed for a huge concrete column.

"That's all I remember, but a week later, when I came out of a coma, I learned that when I smashed head-on into the column, my car had burst into flames. Somehow, I lived through the whole ordeal, but countless bones were broken or pulverized, and I sustained third-degree burns over seventy percent of my body. I couldn't believe I had lived through the collision. I had so wanted to die. Instead, I would have to live through the agonizing pain of a broken body and disfiguring burns.

"I was in the ICU for months, then transferred to a physical rehab, where I learned to walk again and to deal with the excruciating pain. I received a lot of morphine, and after I left rehab six months after the crash, I was hooked. So, three years later, here I am, trying to break my morphine addiction. So far, after a week and a half at ACHIEVE, I haven't felt much progress. I need the goddamned morphine. It's all I have to help me deal with the torture I suffer every fucking moment of my life."

I felt for her. The withdrawal symptoms that I was experiencing couldn't come close to what she was going through. Nevertheless, I was going through one hell of a wicked detox. I remembered my first rehab eight years earlier. Back then, I was given 100 milligrams of Librium every four hours, and the detox went smoothly. I wished I were back there.

I had no appetite, so I excused myself and went to my room to lie down. My heart was pounding, and I felt a huge weight crushing my chest. I stayed in bed until lights out at 10:30. My two roommates came into the room laughing and having themselves a good old time. I envied them. I didn't know how long they had been at ACHIEVE or how severe their withdrawals had been.

After my roommates fell asleep, I relaxed a bit, but I was anxious about having a seizure. It had been more than 48 hours since my last drink, and I was experiencing the textbook symptoms of alcohol withdrawal. Worst of all were the constant tremors, the rapid breathing, and the cold sweats. I also suffered from insomnia, and when I did manage to sleep, I experienced vivid, terrifying nightmares.

The staff continued to check my vitals every two hours. From what I understood, there was no improvement from when I was admitted. I hoped that my numbers would stay high and that they'd have to send me to a hospital to get my blood pressure and pulse rate down. If I were sent there, maybe I'd get some meds to ease my detox. But that didn't happen.

I got through my first night and awoke at 6:30. I looked out the window. It was still dark. I put on a pair of slippers and left my room for the common area. It was empty. I sat on an old, overstuffed couch. My entire body was quivering. I knew it would be at least a few days until my nerves finally settled.

The common area was beginning to fill with patients. On top of a long table were two commercial-sized silver coffee makers, but the last thing I needed was a cup of coffee. As it turned out, all the coffee was decaffeinated, which caused a lot of complaints from patients who wanted their fix. However, I was told that ACHIEVE did not allow caffeine. Too many people were experiencing various degrees of withdrawal, so it was verboten. I'd later learn that even the soft drink vending machine contained only caffeine-free sodas.

Another problem concerned tobacco. There were no cigarettes for sale, but they were allowed if you had them. A couple of people, desperate for real coffee and cigarettes, would sneak out and make a beeline for the convenience store across the street. Most of them got away with it, but those who got caught were discharged from the program. It didn't seem worth the risk to me, but several people didn't want to be there in the first place. Most of them were brought in by family, and a handful were court-ordered. For the court-ordered, it was ACHIEVE or jail.

It was fascinating to watch the people as they returned with their contraband. Every one of these brave, or "I don't give a shit," patients returned with cigarettes, many of which they sold to those who lacked the courage to make the mad dash across the street. Others would return with liters of Coke or Mountain Dew, which I learned packed a lot more caffeine than cola beverages. Others would bring large cups of real coffee.

One girl—her name was Daphne, and she was quite the free spirit—would buy coffee and cigarettes, as well as candy and gum. During the four weeks I was there, five people got caught and kicked out. Daphne got caught once, but for some reason, she was allowed to stay. Even after she was caught, Daphne continued to risk the dangerous trek across the street. She had chutzpah, that was for sure. And she was extremely friendly and kind to everyone, both staff and patients alike. Maybe it was her charm that allowed her to stay after being busted.

Breakfast began at 7:30. I took my place in line and was served by the guy with the shaky hands. We were having waffles, the toaster variety, along with pork sausage links. There was milk and orange juice at the long table against the wall. I filled a glass with juice and grabbed a small carton of milk, then headed to the same group that I sat with the night before—Lucy, Paul, and Gary.

"Still have the shakes, huh?" Paul asked. He was the most talkative and outgoing of the three.

"Yeah," I said, "I know it's going to take a while to get rid of them."

"Just hang in there, buddy. Pretty soon, you'll be as good as new," Paul said.

"What's the deal with the server guy? His hands shake worse than mine," I said.

"Oh, that's Larry. He has five years sober, but he never stops shaking," Paul said. "I had a pretty good talk with him the other day. He really knows his stuff about how alcoholism can fuck you up for good. He told me that forty years of chronic alcoholism affected his nervous system. Something about a Mylar sheath. Anyway, what he said was that he drank more than a fifth of vodka every day for, like I said, forty years. Even after he quit and was sober for over two years, he still had the shakes, mostly in his hands, and his head kind of wobbles, and his voice trembles too. The doctors told him that alcohol eats away at the Mylar, which messes up your nerves. Some people recover, but some, like Larry, will never get rid of the shakes. The damage is just too severe. So, he's stuck with them for the rest of his life. But he's a great guy, and he has a great attitude. He loves being sober."

For the most part, Paul was correct, but what he was calling the Mylar sheath was, in fact, the myelin sheath. Mylar is the foil-like material that's used for shiny party balloons. But myelin is different. It's a crucial component that protects the body's nervous system. Myelin is made up mostly of fat and cholesterol that wrap around the nerve cell to insulate the neuron and direct the nerve's impulse to where it's supposed to go. Alcohol is a solvent, and it eats away at the fatty myelin sheath. When myelin wears down, that opens up a variety of potential problems with memory, movement, and coordination. The shakes are just one of the terrible results of damage to the myelin sheath. Sadly, in Larry's case, that damage was permanent.

"Shit," I said. "If I was going to shake like that the rest of my life, I'm not sure I'd want to quit."

The longest I'd ever been sober was 17 months between Memorial Day of 1987 and October 1988. Even after all that time, my hands had never stopped shaking. I hated eating in front of people or signing my name; my hands shook so badly. After breakfast, I went to my room to lie down. The staff allowed patients who needed more rest to stay in bed for the first day or two. I stayed in bed the entire day, even skipping lunch, so I wouldn't have to interact with anyone. I was just too damn nervous to be around people, and sleep was a phantom I continued to chase. Still, lying in bed alone was better than nothing.

Realizing that I needed nourishment, I dragged myself to the cafeteria for dinner. There was no line. I was the last person to show up. Larry placed two sloppy joes and some fries on my plate. I thanked him, got a glass of juice, and went to sit with the only people I knew.

Lucy was the first to say hello. "We didn't see you in groups today," she said.

"Yeah," I said, "I just stayed in my room trying to get some sleep. That didn't happen, but at least I got some rest. I'll try to make the groups tomorrow."

"Did they give you a schedule?" Lucy asked.

"Yeah, I guess the first group meets at 9:00 tomorrow," I said.

Lucy said, "Some of the groups are pretty good, and at least they help pass the time."

I played with my food and managed to eat one sloppy joe and a few fries.

"Does anyone want my other sandwich?" I asked.

Gary said, "Thanks. I'll take it if you don't want it."

"No. Go ahead; I have no appetite. These damn shakes are killing me."

I got up and said good night. I emptied my tray in the trash and went back to my room to try to sleep. My blood pressure and pulse were still high, and the staff was still monitoring me.

I tossed and turned between staff visits. At 6:00 the next morning, Marlene, one of the health techs, came to my room to take my vitals. My temperature was back to 99 degrees, but my pulse was 110, and my blood pressure was 185 over 100. This was somewhat better than when I first arrived, but she was still concerned. After she left, I got up, walked to the common area, and sat on a couch.

A striking young woman sat next to me. She was drinking what she told me was a cup of instant coffee with real caffeine, and she was smoking a cigarette.

"Hi, my name is Pilar," she said. "You're new, I guess."

"Hi. I'm Rob. I got here the night before last. I'm still shaking pretty bad."

"Alcohol your drug of choice?"

"Yeah. I was in a twenty-eight-day rehab in 1981 at the University of Illinois Hospital, and they gave us Librium until the shaking and danger of seizures were over."

"Yeah, this place is pretty low rent."

"What are you in here for?" I asked.

"Mostly cocaine, and also speed."

"God, I can't even imagine doing any speed right now. Or any time for that matter. I'm way too nervous for that."

"So, I guess you're not interested in a cup of coffee."

"No, thanks. I'm already about to crawl out of my skin."

"Is that why you drink? Because you're so nervous?"

"Yeah, I guess so. When I drink, I'm way more at ease."

"I hardly ever drink," she said. "I can't stand the taste of beer, and I don't like wine much either. Which is good because I'm only nineteen."

"Nineteen, wow. What's the age minimum for this place?" I asked.

"Eighteen. You have to be eighteen to be admitted. I turn twenty next month."

"Well," I said, "Happy Birthday in advance." She didn't ask me how old I was, and that was a good thing. At 33, I felt like a dirty old man.

"Thanks," she said. "So, what will you do with yourself after you stop drinking?"

"I saw a psychiatrist in '83, and he suggested Valium, but I was afraid of getting addicted, so he put me on Inderal, which helped some. Maybe start on some psych meds; I'm not sure."

"That was smart of you to stay away from Valium. I've seen so many doctors, and I've been in a few psych wards. Oh, I want to warn you of the number one drug to stay away from. It's the worst. That's Klonopin. I got so fucking hooked on Klonopin, the withdrawal was hell. But they're not going to be prescribing any meds here anyway. They don't have a license for that."

"Are you on any meds right now?" I asked her.

"No, but the doctors have had me on a bunch of them. Let's see. I've been on Prozac and Paxil; they didn't help at all. You know, I think that the best medication the doctors ever put me on was Wellbutrin. Yeah, I would even consider going back on Wellbutrin if I could kick my fucking cocaine and speed habit. I just love the rush I get when I do coke. I was doing a whole lot before I came in here, probably about three grams a day. But I've been lucky. There's a woman here—Robin—whose septum is fucking destroyed. You'll see her. She usually walks around with Kleenex stuffed up her nostrils because of the constant nosebleeds. One time, I saw her sneeze, and pieces of cartilage flew out of her nose. She's a mess, but she can't stop doing it. I wouldn't be surprised if she was still snorting lines in back of the stage in the cafeteria."

"She's doing coke in here?" I was stunned—and scared. I wanted this to be a safe place. I needed it to be a safe place.

"Oh, you don't know the half of it. People are doing drugs back there, and some are having sex. Don't say you heard it from me, but I know that Robin has fucked at least one other patient. His name is Tony, and he gets her blow. She's married, and her husband even visits her, but she gets high with Tony, and they screw behind the stage."

"Doesn't staff catch on?"

"No, it's like they don't even want to know about all the rule-breaking and shit that goes on around here."

"Well, as long as no one brings in a kegger, I should be safe."

She laughed. "You know, I've been here for almost two weeks, and I haven't seen anyone drinking. Probably because alcohol smells so strong. Anyway, I've gotta go take a shower before breakfast. Remember, when you get out, stay away from Klonopin. It's the drug from hell. Talk to you later. Try to relax, dude."

Pilar knew her shit. She was young, but she was smart.

CHAPTER 25

Hey, Taxi

As my stay at ACHIEVE was drawing to a close, I needed to make plans concerning where I would live after leaving rehab. Kurt had made it clear that I could not move back in with him and Jane, and I didn't blame him.

Fortunately, my new friends, Paul and Gary, had learned of a halfway house in the suburb of Maywood, which is where both my mother and father were born. Room and board were ninety-five dollars a week, and clients were expected to stay for three months. Paul and Gary had already signed up, and I decided to join them.

The halfway house, which was called The New View Inn, was nice, but I was disappointed that I had to share a bedroom. My roommate, Andrew, had been living there for almost a month. He didn't talk much, which was fine by me.

Life at The New View was tightly structured. Each resident had one week to find a job, and we had to be back on the premises by 5:30 for dinner. We also had chores to do, and each week we had to attend three A.A. meetings at the Inn and one outside meeting.

I found a crummy warehouse job in a suburb about five miles away and had to take two buses, then walk the final mile on a road without sidewalks. When the weather was bad, which it often was, I had to maneuver around several large, icy mud puddles.

At the beginning of April, my brother Rick finally paid each of us siblings what he estimated to be our fair share of the house in River Forest that my mother had deeded to him and his wife, Maureen, back in 1980. My mom died of cancer on June 8, 1981. She had been living in a cramped, three-bedroom apartment in Forest Park with the three youngest—Kevin, Kerry, and Kathy. My mother slept on a couch in the living room, which is where she remained until her death. After doing my first 28-day stint at a hospital rehab, I moved in with her and the kids. I had a job at a warehouse and contributed some money, but I had no business sponging off of her when she was so sick. I was a real piece of shit.

I received $4500 from Rick, and I used $3500 to purchase a 1983 Subaru hatchback. It was nothing to look at, but it was reliable transportation and made the commute to work easier.

Within a few weeks of receiving my money, I moved out of the New View and took a job driving a cab as well as a delivery job at Domino's Pizza. Both jobs sucked, especially delivering pizza.

My credit was a joke, so I was unable to rent an apartment. I moved into a Motel 6 that was close to O'Hare. I stayed sober and earned more than enough money to pay the $26 a day for my room and put away some cash.

I quit the Domino's gig and decided to try my luck driving a cab at night. I arrived at the garage at 4:00 p.m. Fred, the dispatcher, said, "You've never driven the night shift before, have you? This will be an experience."

"I bet it will," I said.

"Well, let me give you a bit of advice. You're gonna get a lot of drunks. They can change personalities in a second. Friendly and polite one minute; then, snap, they lose it. Watch yourself; it's crazy out there."

"Thanks," I said, "I'll be careful."

"Well, pick a cab, sign for it. Good luck, and stay safe."

I chose a car that looked okay and headed out to make some money. After leaving the garage, I stopped at a liquor store and bought myself a pint of vodka. I got back in my cab and took a few swigs. I was ready to go.

Most of the fares were fine, but some of the drunks had shitty attitudes. I stayed buzzed and didn't give a fuck. That first night became a blur. I took a few hits of vodka every now and then to maintain my high. At about 10:00 p.m., I picked up a young Black guy and took him to the West Side. We reached his destination, and he paid his fare. I drove off. That was the last thing I remembered about that night.

At 2:30 in the morning, I woke up. I was still in the driver's seat of my cab, but I was parked near Kedzie and Madison, an extremely dangerous locale, especially for a white guy in the wee hours of the morning.

I turned the ignition and got nothing. The radio had likely been playing for hours, and I'd left the headlights on. Now the fucking battery was dead. I left the cab in search of a payphone, and the alcohol gods smiled on me. I found a phone booth, called dispatch, and told them that my battery had died. In about half an hour, a tow truck arrived, and a big, tough-looking guy approached.

"So, your battery's dead? What the hell were you doing around here that drained your battery?"

"I don't know; it just happened."

"Yeah, it just happened," he said.

He gave me a jump, and the cab started right up.

"I suggest you bring the car in for the night," he said.

"Yeah, thanks. Good idea."

He got in his tow truck and drove off.

I drove back to the garage, paid my nut, and learned that I had netted $40. That sucked, but it was my fault. I drove back to the motel and drank some vodka and ginger ale. I watched some TV and fell asleep just before sunrise. I awoke at noon and decided the night shift was not for me. That afternoon, I tried to keep my drinking to a minimum, just enough to keep the shakes at bay. I would go back to the garage in the morning and start over. I awoke at 4:00 a.m., showered, and headed to the garage. When I got there, Fred the dispatcher approached, and he wasn't happy.

"So, what happened the other night?"

"Sorry, I'm not sure how the battery died."

"The tow truck driver said you smelled of alcohol, real strong."

"Really? I don't know why he'd say that. I wasn't drinking."

"Well, I'm gonna give you one more chance. Don't fuck it up. Now go pick a car."

The day dragged on. I bought some vodka, and by two in the afternoon, I'd made $75; my nut was $65. I decided my time was worth more than ten bucks a day. So, I drove the cab to a spot next to the garage, left the keys on the driver's seat, and walked to my car. I was out of the cab driving and pizza business in the blink of an eye. I didn't have the money to pay for the motel and began living in my car.

I got in touch with Paul, whose roommate had started drinking again and moved out. Paul let me detox in the guy's former bedroom. After three days, I had arranged for another stay at ACHIEVE. They had a payment plan that let me give $100 upfront and make payments after my release. Paul lent me the $100 and drove me to ACHIEVE.

When I got out of rehab, I began driving a cab for a company in the northwest suburbs. Jeff, another friend from the New View, lent me the money for my first week's nut, which was $200. The cab was mine twenty-four-seven as long as I paid my weekly nut.

After my first four days, I had netted more than $500. I paid Paul and Jeff, moved out of Paul's apartment, and got a room at another Motel 6. This one was in Elk Grove Village. As long as I stayed sober, I made good money. I worked six days a week, fourteen hours a day, and was bringing home $1000 a week.

I made friends with another cab driver, Herb Sorenson, who owned a condo in the adjoining suburb of Wood Dale. Like me, Herb enjoyed his beer—too much. I rented his basement for sixty dollars a week, and as long as I stayed sober, I did just fine. However, within a few months, I was drinking each night after work and every weekend.

CHAPTER 26

The Pancreas Strikes Back

Although I was drinking more than I should, I was working regularly, paying Herb on time, and I was satisfied with my accommodations. My basement apartment beat the hell out of the flophouses and SROs I'd occupied in San Diego and on Chicago's Near North Side.

Then, all hell broke loose. At 4:00 on the Monday morning of April 5, 1993, my body could no longer withstand its daily assault of alcohol. As I shakily attempted to shave a three-day growth of beard without separating my head from my torso, my stomach burned like never before. I stumbled to the fridge, pressing my hand hard against my gut, and found a bottle of Maalox. I took a few swigs and went back to the bathroom to wait for the Maalox to start working. But the pain grew worse, and I puked the milky white liquid all over the sink and mirror. I shaved as quickly as I could and went back for more Maalox. The dose lasted until midway through my shower. At least this mess went straight down the drain.

I found some Tums, took a few, and went back to bed in my wet towel. I was very thirsty, so I took some water from a glass on the nightstand. I felt like someone was slashing my gut with a dull, rusty knife. Next, an intense pain began radiating from my abdomen to my lower back. I pushed out my stomach as far as I could to try to ease the back pain. Then, I puked. I drank more water, and I puked again. I was burning up with a thirst I couldn't quench. Every sip of water I took came right back up.

I lay in bed throughout the day, drenched in sweat, vomiting constantly, and wiping the detritus from my mouth and chin. At about 4:30 that afternoon, I could hear Herb's footsteps upstairs. I managed to put on some clothes and struggled upstairs.

"Gee, Rob," Herb said, "you look terrible. What's the matter?"

"I don't know, but my stomach and back are killing me. Could you please give me a ride to the hospital?"

"Sure thing, Rob. Boy, you don't look good. I'll get you there right away."

"Thanks, Herb," I said.

I made my way to his cab and sat in the back. I hoped I wouldn't throw up in his car.

"Well, Rob, Alexian Brothers is the nearest hospital. Or, if you'd like, I could drive you to Elmhurst Hospital. Do you have a preference?"

I wanted to scream, "*Just get me to a fucking hospital,*" but I merely groaned. "Alexian Brothers is good," I said. "Please hurry."

We reached the hospital in ten minutes.

"Well, here we are, Rob. Do you need some help getting inside?"

I knew he wanted to get the hell out of there, so I told him no, thanks, I could make it on my own.

"Gee, okay, Rob. Good luck. I hope they can help you."

The moment I got inside, a nurse saw how bad off I was, and they immediately placed me in a wheelchair and brought me to an examination room. The nurse and a patient tech helped me onto a bed. Almost instinctively, the nurse handed me one of those pink tubs, the ones they keep for the heavy barfers. Her timing was impeccable, and I immediately began retching and vomiting. The barf splashed everywhere.

Two men entered the room. "Hello, Mr. Rickelman." A tall, slightly overweight man wearing green scrubs spoke first. He was likely about forty and sported recently trimmed, dark brown hair.

"I'm Doctor Carbon, and this is Doctor Vincente. We understand you're experiencing severe abdominal pain. Can you describe it for us?"

"It's mostly my belly just above my navel. It feels like I'm being sliced open. My back is killing me, and I can't hold anything down, not even a sip of water."

"Stomach distended," Dr. Carbon said.

"Yes, and cyanosis. His lips are blue," Dr. Vincente replied. "Let's get some blood drawn."

He left for a moment and quickly returned. Within minutes, a man in blue scrubs arrived and swabbed an area of skin around a vein on the back of my hand. He tied an elastic band around my upper arm and inserted a needle into my vein. He filled three vials with blood, then removed the needle and asked me to keep my arm raised for a bit. He thanked me and left.

Dr. Carbon addressed me. "Would you pull up your shirt, please?"

I did as I was told, and he jabbed a finger into my belly, just above the navel.

I moaned. "God, it hurts like hell."

"Acute pancreatitis," said Dr. Carbon.

"Yeah, pain radiating from mid-belly, major back pain." Dr. Vincente said.

Dr. Vincente held my wrist and looked at his watch.

"His pulse is racing. I've got 127." He sounded concerned.

Dr. Vincente stuck a thermometer in my ear. It quickly beeped, and he announced, "He has a high fever, 103.9."

He turned to a nurse and said, "Let's give him 100 milligrams of Demerol. See how he does with that."

Dr. Carbon looked up from his notes. "Are you a heavy drinker, Mr. Rickelman?"

"Yes, I'm an alcoholic."

"When was your last drink?"

"Yesterday afternoon."

"How much did you consume?"

"Yesterday? Just beer, about a case."

"And is that a typical daily amount?"

"I, I guess so. Sometimes I drink more, sometimes a little less. I drink a lot of vodka too."

As the doctors turned away, two burly guys in scrubs entered. They were patient techs, and they did the heavy lifting, transporting, and clean-up of patients.

"Hi, Robert," one said. "My name's Tony, and this is Ron. We're gonna get you changed out of those messy clothes and into a nice fresh gown."

They were good at what they did, effortlessly rolling me on my side, lifting me, getting rid of my crusty clothes, and into a clean gown. They were very kind.

"There you go. Are you a bit more comfortable now?"

"Yes," I whispered. "Thank you."

"It's our job to keep you comfortable and safe. If you need anything, just press the nurse's button." He motioned to a button on the bed rail.

"We'll be in and out to make sure you're doing okay."

The nurse had left and returned to my room. She hung a bag of clear fluids from a tall steel pole. She deftly inserted an IV needle into a vein on my upper right forearm and secured it with a few strips of tape.

"This bag contains electrolytes and glucose. I also have something for pain," she said.

She administered the Demerol by pushing a syringe into an access port attached to the IV. Then, she connected another line to a different access port. That line was connected to a piggyback bag, which contained an antibiotic.

I felt a warm, slightly stinging sensation, but I didn't mind. I expected relief to follow, but almost immediately, I was puking forcefully into the pink tub. My gown was an ugly mess, splattered with globs of dark brown, green, and yellow.

"I'll ask the doctor for something for nausea," the nurse said.

She turned and left.

My room was the hub of ER activity that late afternoon.

The nurse appeared with another syringe.

"This is Compazine. It's for nausea, and it's going to make you sleepy."

Once again, she placed a syringe into the port and pushed the contents through.

"How is your pain?" she asked.

"It's really bad," I said.

"I'll talk to the doctor." She left again.

For the first time, I had a moment to reflect on what was taking place. I correctly surmised that my condition was serious. I was disappointed that the shot of Demerol was not easing my pain. Just then, the nurse returned. I saw the syringe in her right hand; I hoped it was more Demerol.

"The doctor wants me to give you an extra 50 milligrams of the Demerol. Combined with the 100 we gave you a short time ago, that's a very high dose. You should get some relief now."

The 150 milligrams began to lessen the pain. And with the Compazine, the nausea was subsiding.

Dr. Carbon was back. "How's your pain?" he asked.

"I have some, but it's nothing like before," I said.

"You'll be NPO for a while. That means nothing by mouth. You'll receive all your fluids and nutrients intravenously."

"Can I drink water?"

"Absolutely not. You can't even have ice chips."

"We've also started you on Cipro, which is an antibiotic. You're going to undergo a battery of tests—an MRI, CT scan, and an ultrasound. We'll know after these tests whether your pancreas is necrotic. That means that some, we can't yet say how much, of your pancreatic tissue is dead. This could result in infection or worse, gangrene. But, as I said, we won't know anything until we do the tests. You're going to be with us for the next several days."

As he turned to leave, he delivered some much-needed good news. "I'll have the nurse give you more pain and nausea meds. She will be inserting a tube—a nasogastric tube, or NG—through one of your nostrils to your stomach. We need to suction the toxic and corrosive enzymes from your stomach. It will be a rather unpleasant procedure."

"Doctor," I asked, "what about my liver?"

"Oh, don't worry about your liver," he said. "Your pancreas is going to kill you first." I think he smiled when he said that.

I remained at the hospital for thirteen days. The NG tube—which, by the way, was inserted with a good deal of discomfort—stayed in place for eight days. I received my first ice chips the day the NG tube was removed. On my tenth day, I was placed on a liquid diet, and the day before I was released, I began eating soft foods such as Jello and yogurt.

The hospital staff had saved my life and facilitated my recovery.

I was grateful for their care. After I was released, I managed to stay sober for six months. Then, I backslid to what I did best—drinking heavily and nursing hangovers.

CHAPTER 27

December DUI

By December of 1994, I was drinking daily and leasing a cab from Marco, a very nice guy who had been a high school math teacher in Mexico. That was the funny thing about cab drivers; the foreign guys were often professionals in their native country who weren't deemed qualified to fill their old positions in the U.S. Almost all the foreign guys drove seven days a week, 12 hours a day.

On the other hand, if you were white and were not a student working your way through college, you had almost certainly fucked up somewhere along the way and found yourself driving a hack. If you weren't an actively drinking alcoholic, you were in "recovery," which meant you were trying to stay sober.

I was driving nights. It was about two in the morning, and I had just dropped off two scary-looking guys after taking them to make a crack buy. When you drive at night, you take what you can get. As it turned out, these guys were okay, and they gave me a nice tip.

I headed to an all-night Osco and bought a liter of Listerine. I drank enough to catch a nice buzz and was feeling okay.

However, driving a cab while drinking Listerine has its drawbacks. After taking a few drunks home from the local taverns, I took that one slug too many. The next thing I knew, there was a hard rapping on my driver's window. It was a cop; two actually. It seems that I had smashed my cab into a parked motorcycle and buried the bike in a four-foot snowdrift. It was 3:36 a.m. I was drunk as hell, but I remember it was 3:36.

"Sir, are you all right?" one of the cops asked.

My brain was stuffed with sticky, menthol, cotton candy. I lifted my head slowly off the steering wheel.

"Huh? What? Where am I?" Not exactly what you want an officer to hear when you're sitting behind the wheel.

"Sir, please step out of the car."

"Oooh! Yeah. Just a second, please," I said. I tried not to slur.

I opened the door and stumbled out.

"Sir, have you been drinking? Are you intoxicated?"

"Yes, officer. I've had a little something to drink."

I think they laughed. I would have.

The cops were bundled up against the frigid air. One of them produced a breathalyzer.

"Sir, I'm going to need you to blow into this breathalyzer."

"I only live a half-block away. Can't I just go home?" I was telling the truth. Instead of turning onto my street, I had drunkenly steered into the parking lot of another apartment complex and plowed the motorcycle into the snowbank. The bike was barely visible.

"I'm sorry, sir. You appear to be extremely intoxicated. You'll need to stay here with us."

"Okay, officer. Sure. What do you need again?"

"I have a breathalyzer here, sir. We need you to blow into it."

I did as I was told.

He showed the breathalyzer to his partner.

"Sir, it's obvious that you are severely intoxicated. You've just registered a .236. That's an extreme DUI."

He tried to show me the breathalyzer, but I was seeing two of everything, and couldn't focus on the little red digits.

"Sir, we are placing you under arrest. You're going with us to the station."

"But what about the cab? We can't just leave it here; it's not even mine. I just live a half a block away. Is it okay if I just drive it home?

I was standing in a pool of antifreeze.

"The car will be fine, sir. We'll have it towed."

"But I have to give it back to my friend at 5:00."

"I'm sorry, sir, but you're coming with us. Please put your hands behind your back."

I obliged, and the handcuffs clicked behind me. One of the officers opened the rear passenger door, and I got in. It was a short drive to the station. We parked in a lot with all the other cruisers, and the officer who cuffed me opened the door to let me out. We entered the station through a rear entrance.

The officer uncuffed me and led me to a small cell. There was a steel bed attached to the wall at about waist height. It had an inch-thick plastic mat that measured about six feet by maybe two and a half.

The stainless steel sink was part of a one-piece multipurpose plumbing apparatus. In other words, the drinking fountain was attached to the toilet. I knew I was fucked, and would probably never drive a cab again. I took a seat at the edge of what I hoped wouldn't be my bed for the night. I was only in my cell for 15 or 20 minutes when one of the officers came to the door.

"Robert, please come with me. We're going to get your fingerprints and a couple of photos."

So, they printed me and took my mug shot. The longer I was at the police station, the more the booze was wearing off.

A big bald cop, a sergeant with gray eyes the color of his mustache, and a bit too heavy to chase down a criminal, spoke.

"Robert, I have some good news. We're going to let you go on an "I" bond, which in lawyer-talk is a personal recognizance bond. To put it simply, you're going to sign this paper, where you agree to appear in court on the date scheduled. Your date is January 3, 1995. If you don't show up, the judge is gonna issue a warrant for your arrest, and you'll be in a bigger bag of shit than you already are. Do you understand that, Robert?"

"Yes, Sergeant," I said.

"Okay, then we have a deal. Just sign here, and you get to sleep in your own bed. Our officers will drive you home."

"Thank you, Sergeant," I said as I signed the paper.

"Billy, Mike, would you be so kind as to drive Mr. Rickelman home?"

"No problem, Sarge. Right this way, Robert."

I didn't know if it was Billy or Mike addressing me. I just knew I was going home to a nice bottle of vodka, to forget this for at least a few hours. Marco was going to be mighty upset.

We left through the rear and I got in the car. The three of us were silent for a ride that lasted less than five minutes. They let me out on the street in front of my parking lot.

"Don't forget, Robert, January 3. And if I were you, I'd get some help with that drinking," an officer said.

"Thanks, officers. I promise, no more drinking for me." *At least not until I get inside.*

As they slowly drove away, I knew I'd lost another round to my nemesis, Mr. John Barleycorn. *Well played, Mr. Barleycorn. Well played.*

CHAPTER 28

Down on My Luck in a Basement Apartment

The cops dropped me off, and I went inside; it was 4:45 a.m. I poured myself a tumbler of vodka and drank it straight. I would need a good buzz to call Marco and tell him I'd wrecked his car.

At 5:00 a.m., after slamming down my vodka, I called him with the bad news. He sounded stunned and upset, but even though I'd totally screwed him, he didn't lash out. His lack of anger made me feel even worse for what I'd done. After that phone call, I lay on my bed and wondered what in the hell I was going to do with a DUI hanging over my head and no means of income. I checked my stash—I didn't even have a bank account—and counted all the money I had to my name. My net worth was $900.

I had been paying Herb Sorenson sixty bucks each week to live in his basement. I had no stove or refrigerator, but he let me use his. I usually ate at fast food joints, and I rarely kept anything in his fridge. I also used his bathroom and shower, but I always kept my beer and vodka downstairs with me, and I was accustomed to drinking them piss-warm.

I knew that Herb would be awake already, and I lay low while I listened to his footsteps. I drifted off to sleep and woke just after

9:00 a.m. I knew that Marco had probably already told the cab company about his car, and I knew that Herb would soon be aware of what had occurred.

I checked the Yellow Pages for DUI lawyers and realized that there was no way I could afford to pay an attorney. I didn't even know how much longer I could pay my rent. I needed a job immediately, probably at a warehouse or a factory. But I was drinking 24 hours a day and was in no condition to search for a job. Besides, I didn't even own a car. I was fucked, and I stayed in the basement all day and all night long, only venturing out for the mile-long walk to Osco to stock up on beer. There was no sidewalk, just an ice and snow-covered parkway that I was forced to navigate.

Christmas passed with me drinking alone in my basement hideaway, and my January 3 court date soon arrived. I called a taxi to get to the DuPage County Courthouse in Wheaton, which was fifteen miles away. I was dressed in a pair of gray slacks and a white dress shirt hidden under a dark green parka. The cab cost me over thirty bucks each way, which cut deeply into my savings.

I found my assigned courtroom and took a seat to wait for my case to be called. I had not drunk any alcohol that morning, and I was a bundle of nerves. I had decided to plead guilty, which meant that my license would be suspended for six months. When my case was called, I approached the bench, and the judge asked me where my lawyer was. I told him that I didn't have a lawyer and that I wanted to plead guilty, which was my right to do. But this pompous, asshole judge went off on me.

"How dare you come to my courtroom without an attorney?" he demanded. "I should hold you in contempt of court right here and now, but I'm going to continue your case to Tuesday, January 31, and you had better have a lawyer with you."

I stood before him, trembling both from fear and severe

alcohol withdrawal. I just wanted out of there. I went to the clerk for a copy of the continuance. I understood enough about the law to know that the judge did not have the right to make me hire a lawyer, but I was physically and mentally in no condition to challenge him.

I left the courthouse, jumped into a cab, and had the driver stop at a liquor store where I bought two cases of beer. When I got home, I got plastered while I tried to sort things out. I knew that I was never setting foot in that courthouse again, but as for my alternatives, all I could do was stay good and drunk.

The days passed, and I continued my drinking unabated. January 31 arrived, and I skipped my court date. That must have pissed off that fucking judge. *Screw him*, I thought. But I was almost out of money, and having my alcohol was much more important than spending sixty bucks on a round-trip to the courthouse.

By Monday, February 13, I had no money, no food, and no beer. Two days later, Herb knocked on my door and told me that I couldn't live in his basement rent-free. I didn't know what to do.

I stayed in the basement for a few more days. The withdrawals were merciless, but after three days, I had weathered the worst of them. I spent the next seven days without a bite of food. On February 23, I called my brother Kurt and told him of my predicament He was ticked off that I had drunk myself into another hole I couldn't climb out of. He called my brother Ray, who was living in Tucson. Thankfully, Ray offered to pay for a one-way flight for me to come out to Arizona and get my shit together. On Friday evening, February 24, my brother Rick came to fetch me, and I said goodbye to Herb. He was glad to see me go, and I didn't blame him.

I spent Friday night at Rick and Maureen's house in River Forest. The following morning, Rick dropped me at Kurt and

Jane's house in Oak Park. I weighed myself on their bathroom scale and was not surprised to see that my weight had dropped to 152 pounds. I was 5'11" and my weight was the same as when I'd stayed at the 13th and Island detox in San Diego.

On Sunday morning, February 26, Kurt drove me to the airport, and we said farewell. I was going to miss him and Rick, but I was grateful to get the hell out of Illinois.

CHAPTER 29

Moving to Tucson

I boarded the plane, found my seat, and settled in. I was anxious as hell. I wanted to order a drink, but I didn't have a penny to my name. I knew that was a good thing.

We landed in Tucson shortly after noon. As I stepped off the jetway, I spotted Ray and my niece, Kaitlin. Ray was smiling—I was glad to see that—and three-and-a-half-year-old Kaitlin was eating Kix cereal from a zip-lock bag. It felt good to be in Tucson. We walked to the baggage pickup, then headed outside. The warm sun felt wonderful—a welcome change from Chicago's frigid weather.

We arrived at Ray's house. Ray had converted the den into a bedroom with a full-size bed, a dresser, and a TV. He was going out of his way to make me comfortable, and I appreciated all he had done. It was up to me to stay sober and turn my life around. As I unpacked my clothes, I found two twenty-dollar bills stuffed into a rolled-up pair of socks. I would have killed to have come across forty bucks while I was detoxing in that basement in Wood Dale. I didn't say a word about my sudden windfall, but I had a sneaking suspicion that the money I'd found would mean nothing but trouble.

At the end of my second week in Arizona, it was time to find a job. I did not want to live with Ray and his family for too long. I checked the Sunday classifieds and decided to apply for a patient transport position at Saint Joseph Hospital, which was about five miles from Ray's house.

At 1:30 on Monday afternoon, I placed an orange ten-speed bicycle in the bed of Ray's blue Ford pick-up truck, and he dropped me near the hospital. I slung a lock and chain over my shoulder and removed the bike. I thanked Ray for the ride, and he drove away.

I had the forty dollars in my pocket, and I was feeling incredibly anxious and uneasy. Instead of taking the parkway that led to the hospital, I pedaled south on Wilmot Road in search of a store to buy a bottle of Listerine. When I reached Broadway, I turned east and spotted a Walgreens. I turned into the parking lot, locked my bike, and went inside. I paid three dollars for two six-ounce bottles, which I stuffed into my pants pockets. I headed to the hospital.

After locking the bike to a rack, I entered the building and found a men's room. I ducked into a stall and quickly downed the two bottles. The Listerine burned, and I felt nauseated, but I knew that would pass when the alcohol kicked in.

Within a few minutes, I started to feel the Listerine's effect. I thought the buzz was too much and felt discernibly tipsy. Nevertheless, I found the human resources department and told the receptionist that I wanted to apply for the transporter position. I wondered if she could tell I was drunk.

She handed me an application, and I filled it out. My handwriting was barely legible, but I turned it in and asked when I would be interviewed. She said that they were not interviewing that day and that if they were interested, they would phone me, which they never did.

By the time I left and reached my bike, my alcohol buzz had intensified. I was sure I would be busted if I showed up at Ray's in my current condition. I decided to take a long, meandering route to afford myself some time to sober up. At one point, I stopped at a 7-Eleven and bought two instant lottery tickets. Maybe I'd hit it big and not have to give a shit about being drunk. I scratched both cards and, of course, they were losers, just like me. I pedaled home, hoping that my indiscretion would go unnoticed.

Fortunately, things were busy at the house, with Ray, Therese, and the three kids, Whitney, Brad, and Kaitlin, all at home. It was just after four, and my alcohol buzz was gradually diminishing. Everyone seemed too distracted to notice the hint of Listerine on my breath. Besides, no one there had any inclination that Listerine used to be my go-to when I was working for Alex Galvin.

At 5:00, we had dinner—Stouffer's lasagna—which was pretty tasty. Ray drank his usual two bottles of Heineken, and Therese enjoyed a couple of glasses of wine. Therese asked me how my job search had gone, and I answered that the St. Joe's job looked promising. That was a whopper.

After dinner, I did the dishes, and as I stood at the sink, I relaxed, certain that there was too much alcohol in the air for my fading Listerine breath to raise any eyebrows. When I finished the dishes, Ray and I watched the news in the living room while Therese worked on her laptop. We watched TV until 8:00 when I told Ray that I was bushed, and I went to bed. Once in my room, I couldn't believe how stupid I had been for drinking that Listerine.

I awoke at 7:30 Tuesday morning and went into the kitchen for a glass of water. Therese had left for work, and Whitney and Brad were at school. I was feeling extremely nervous and was craving a drink, but Ray had the day off from work, and he had kept Kaitlin home from daycare.

I tried to steer clear of Ray; I didn't want him to see how edgy I was. Then, I received some good news. Ray was going to Ace Hardware, and he wanted to know if I'd like to join him. I declined his invitation and was relieved when he said that he was taking Kaitlin.

As soon as Ray pulled out of the driveway, I went to the refrigerator to look for beer. To my disappointment, there was none in the fridge. I knew that Therese liked to keep wine on hand. I rummaged through the pantry and found two unopened bottles of chardonnay on a lower shelf. I knew that I was making a decision there would be no coming back from. I grabbed a corkscrew and opened the first bottle, which I emptied in less than five minutes. I opened the second bottle, and I quickly downed it.

I filled both bottles with water, replaced the corks, and positioned their wrinkled gold foil over the necks. It was a half-assed job, and I knew that this switcheroo would be readily detected, but I was desperate. I hurried to the bathroom to shower and brush my teeth.

As I was leaving the bathroom, I almost walked right into Ray. I nearly jumped out of my skin. Ray asked if I was okay, and I told him I was fine, just a bit startled. I went into my bedroom to dress. I checked the pockets of the pants I'd worn to the hospital the day before and was relieved to count $35—a twenty, a ten, and five singles. That was plenty of money to get good and drunk on.

I could hear Ray in the hall, and I wondered how I was going to hide the fact that I'd just killed two bottles of wine. I was feeling drunker by the minute. Then, Ray shouted that he'd bought the wrong size screw, and he'd have to return to the Ace.

Please take Kaitlin. Please take Kaitlin, I prayed.

My prayers were answered when Ray called to me that he was taking Kaitlin with him.

The moment he left, I went to the garage to retrieve the bicycle and chain from the day before. I wasn't sure what I was going to do, but I knew that I had to get away. I biked through the neighborhood until I reached a nearby 7-Eleven. I went inside without locking the bike and bought a six-pack of Budweiser. I asked the clerk to double-bag it and left the store.

Ray's house was less than a block from a large wash called East Arroyo Chico, which was bordered on both sides by thick oleander bushes that probably rose twenty feet high. It was the perfect place to hide out and drink my beer, so I rode there and found a secluded spot. I was going to get plastered, and nothing would get in my way.

I lay the bike on the ground and popped open my first beer. I drank these beers slowly and relished every sip. It was 9:45; I had the entire day to stay leisurely drunk, and the money to do it. I counted my cash; I had thirty dollars and some change.

By noon, the beer was gone. I decided to tour Tucson. I carried the bike out of the wash and pedaled back to Tucson Boulevard. I took a right to Broadway and cycled west to the intersection where Campbell Avenue became Kino Parkway, which was named for the Italian-born, Spanish Jesuit missionary Eusebio Francisco Kino, who, in 1692, arrived in the area that would become Tucson.

I traveled south on Kino Parkway, and at the northwest corner of the intersection of Kino and 15th Street, I came upon the magnificent bronze statue of Padre Kino on horseback. I gently placed my bike on the ground to gaze at the statue. I had seen it briefly when Ray drove me to his house from the airport. Ray spoke to me of the many accomplishments of Padre Kino, and I had been duly impressed. I thought about how he had sailed from Europe, reached and explored New Spain, and founded so many missions, and there I was, drunk and jobless on a road to nowhere.

After admiring that statue, I got back on my bike and crossed the parkway where 15th Street became Winsett. The area was filled with factories and warehouses, and I decided to do some exploring.

After riding southeast for a block, I was surprised to come upon a second, smaller Campbell Avenue, less impressive than the first, but an interesting find, nonetheless.

I turned right on that Campbell and pedaled slowly south until, on my right just before 19th Street, I caught sight of the Alcoholics Anonymous Central Office. It was an unassuming, one-story, red-brick building with a green awning and door; two cars were parked next to the place. Spotting the site where A.A. operations throughout Tucson were overseen was unnerving. There I was, smack dab in front of A.A. headquarters, drunk as a lord in the middle of the day. I felt guilty and hypocritical. *Fuck you, A.A.*, I thought as I turned my bike around and headed back toward Winsett.

I wanted to find a dark tavern where I could day drink alongside my alcoholic brethren, but I doubted that I would find such an oasis in that industrial park. To my delight, when I reached Plumer Avenue, I spied a nondescript, dull-gray building with quite a few cars and a couple of motorcycles parked in front. I chained my bike to a street light pole and locked it. The bar was called The Gray Matter Watering Hole. The irony of entering a place that presented a danger to my own gray matter was not lost on me.

I walked inside. No one acknowledged me as I sidled up to the bar and sat on an old wooden stool with a cracked leather seat. The bartender approached me, and I ordered a Budweiser and a shot of Southern Comfort. He turned to fetch my order, set the drinks in front of me, and said, "That'll be three dollars and fifty cents."

I gave him the twenty, and he returned with my change. I looked at a clock on the wall; it was 1:15. Time was moving slowly, and the bar was silent as a shadow. Each patron wanted to be left alone with their drink, and I relished the gloomy vibe.

By 4:00, I'd drunk five shots and the same number of beers, and I was very drunk. I didn't want to get thrown out of the place, so I plunked down a tip and left without saying a word. I reached my bike feeling very tipsy. I had ten dollars left, and I didn't want to go back to Ray's house. So, I unlocked my bike and rode on. I was much drunker than the night before, but I focused on pedaling safely and headed in the general direction of Ray's place.

Rush hour traffic was getting heavy, and I maneuvered my bicycle with some difficulty. I reached Broadway and Kino, entered a Safeway supermarket, and spent seven dollars on a pint of cheap vodka and a liter of Sprite. Dusk was falling as I left the store and headed back to the spot in the arroyo where my journey had begun.

I settled into the arroyo, opened the Sprite, and poured half of the bottle into the sandy soil. I unscrewed the cap of the vodka bottle and carefully drained it into the green bottle of Sprite. Despite being extremely intoxicated, I managed not to spill a drop. I took a long pull from the bottle, and that was the last thing I remembered.

The next thing I knew, it was daytime, and I was in a hospital bed hooked up to a ventilator with an IV in my arm. Ray and Therese were at my bedside. I had no clue as to what had transpired or how long I'd been in the hospital.

When I saw the pained look on Ray's face, a tear rolled down my cheek. Therese looked concerned but calm.

"Well," Ray said, "you're finally awake."

"Where am I?" I asked.

"You're at the University Medical Center," Ray said. "You got here early last night, around 7:00. Some guy was walking his dog, and he noticed you unconscious in the wash. The cops and paramedics arrived. Brad heard the sirens and walked to the arroyo to see what was going on. He watched them put you on a stretcher and into an ambulance.

"He was so shaken up, he ran home yelling, 'There's something wrong with Uncle Rob. They took him away in an ambulance. I think he's dead.'"

Therese admonished me. "It was a terrible thing for him to see. He's only fourteen."

Ray asked, "Do you know how lucky you are that that guy happened to pass by? You would have died in that wash. They had to pump your stomach, and then they intubated you."

"What time is it?" I asked.

"It's 11:00 a.m. You've been in a coma for 16 hours. How could you do this to yourself? We try to help you, and you just turn around and throw it all away."

I didn't know what to say. Thankfully, at that moment, a pretty young nurse entered the room.

"Well, good morning, Robert, I'm so glad you're awake. My name is Diane. From what I've been told, it was pretty much touch and go with you last night."

I began to gag on the large tube that ran to my lungs. I struggled to talk, and the nurse told me to take some deep breaths and relax. She handed me a small pad of paper and a felt marker.

"Here you go," the nurse said, "if you have any questions, you can just jot them down."

The first thing I wrote was, "When can you remove the breathing tube?"

"Well," she said, "that's a good question. We'll probably keep the tube in until you are more alert and able to breathe on your own. It'll probably be an hour or two."

My next question was when I would be released.

She laughed. "Someone's not fond of our accommodations. Well, right now you're in our Intensive Care Unit. If things go well, and we remove the tube, you'll probably go to the immediate care unit, and then you'll be placed in a regular room for another day or two. After that, let's say Friday, you'll be released. How does that sound?"

I smiled and whispered, "Thank you."

"You are very welcome. I'll be close by if you need anything. Just relax and concentrate on getting better." She turned and left.

When the nurse was gone, Therese said, "You know, Rob, it's not a good idea for you to stay with us. Brad was terrified of what he saw, and we just can't risk another incident."

She was protecting her brood, and I could appreciate that. Therese's maternal instincts notwithstanding, I was staring homelessness square in the face.

Ray said, "Well, we'll let you get some rest. I'll check on you tomorrow." And with that, he and Therese were gone.

I was glad to see them go. I needed to rest, and Therese's pronouncement that I would not be living with them was a daunting, though not unexpected, bit of news. I didn't know anything about Tucson, and the only prospects I could envision were shelters or homelessness.

At 11:45, Diane stopped in and checked my ventilator tube. "Your breathing seems to be good. Let's see if we can get the doctor to okay removing this."

At 12:30, she returned with a CNA. "I have some good news, Robert. The doctor said that we can extubate you. We're going to disconnect the ventilator. Oh . . . and I'm sorry. We'll also need to remove your catheter."

She introduced the CNA. "Robert, this is Lucinda. She's going to help remove things."

I managed to smile and nodded toward Lucinda. She smiled back. Then they went to work. Lucinda fetched a large plastic tub, and Diane removed the tape that was securing the tubing. Once the tape was removed, Diane said, "Okay, Robert, I need you to relax and breathe slowly. I'm going to remove the tubing. This might be a bit uncomfortable."

She then began slowly, smoothly pulling the tubing from inside my mouth. I fought the urge to gag as Diane removed it. Lucinda placed the tubing in the bucket, and I took a deep breath.

"Now, we just need to remove your catheter."

They worked quickly; it stung like hell, but I was soon free of all the tubing.

"Okay, we're finished," Diane said. "That wasn't so bad, was it?"

"No, you were both great. Thank you so much," I said. My throat was raw, and my voice was hoarse. "Do you think I could have some ice water?" I asked.

"Absolutely," Diane said. "And later we'll give you some Jell-O and maybe some broth. If that goes well, you'll probably be moved to the next ward. Oh, and before I forget, the doctor ordered 50 milligrams of a sedative to help you with any alcohol withdrawal. It's called Librium, and it's quite effective. It will help take the edge off."

My heart glowed at the good news.

"Thank you so much," I said. "I sure could use something for my nerves."

The two women left, and Diane returned with a plastic pitcher of ice water. She poured me a glass, and it tasted wonderful. Then she handed me a small plastic cup with two white and green capsules. This was the Librium. I took it gratefully.

"Okay, then, Robert, we'll give the medication some time to work, and I'll drop in soon to check on you," she said.

Later that afternoon, I ate the Jell-O and drank the broth. Diane told me that if I had no bad reaction, they would prepare to move me. I would be sorry to lose Diane. She was so charming and kind.

At 3:00, she arrived to tell me that I would be moving to the immediate care ward. By 3:15, an orderly arrived to move me to a new room. I didn't get a chance to thank Diane or say goodbye.

The orderly wheeled my bed to a large elevator, and we went up a few floors. He found my room and wheeled my bed next to a window. I had a roommate—an old guy—but he was asleep. Once I was settled in, I watched a little TV.

I managed to doze off. I awoke to the phone ringing, and I answered it. It was Ray calling to see how I was doing.

"Hey, Ray," I said. "I had something to eat, and they moved me to a new ward. I'm feeling pretty good."

"That's great, Rob, but I'm worried about what we're gonna do with you when you get released. I heard of a detox center near Grant and Alvernon. I'll try to get you admitted there when you leave UMC. After that, I'm not sure what we're gonna do. But I just wanted to let you know that I'm working on it."

"Thanks, Ray," I said. "I don't deserve a brother like you. I'm so sorry I screwed up."

"Well, that's water under the bridge. We just have to move on. Now, get some rest. I'll call you tomorrow."

"Hey, Ray," I said. "I want you to know I love you and I appreciate all you've done for me. Sorry, I'm such a mess."

"I love you, too. Gotta go." Ray was not the sentimental type, but I knew he loved me.

I was receiving the Librium every six hours, and the next day, I was moved to a regular ward. At 11:00 Friday morning, I was released from the hospital. Ray was there to pick me up. I wondered how I was going to do without my Librium.

"Okay," Ray said as we walked out of the hospital, "I got you into that detox place I was talking about. It's called Nueva Vista. Let's get going."

We drove a couple of miles to a fair-sized complex of one-story buildings. Ray parked his truck and retrieved a small bag of clothes he'd chosen for me. We approached the door, and Ray rang a buzzer. A young man, probably in his late twenties, opened the door and let us in.

Ray spoke first. "Hi, I called to get a spot for my brother to get help with his detox." He motioned to me.

"Well, first of all, let me introduce myself," the man said. "My name is Tim, and I'm one of the nurses. And you must be Robert," he said to me. I nodded my head.

"We're a seven-day detox and rehab center. Most of our patients are suffering from alcoholism, but we do have some who are trying to quit other drugs. We're always busy, and there are four patients to each room. We have one section for men and another for women."

"Is this a medical detox?" I asked.

"Sadly, no," Tim said. "We're not licensed for that. So some of our patients have a pretty rough go of it. We're fairly close to the Tucson Medical Center, and there's a fire station nearby. So, if anyone experiences any difficulties, help is close by. And, of course, we have nurses and nurses' aides."

"But no doctors?" I asked.

"Sorry, no doctors. But you'll be in good hands. And we don't charge our patients to stay here. The state of Arizona covers that."

I did not like his answers at all. I wanted some fucking Librium.

"Well," Ray said to me, "it looks like you're in good hands, Rob, so I'm gonna get going. I'll talk to you soon."

I wanted to go with him, but that was not an option. I would be at the fucking Nueva Vista for the next several days. Ray hugged me and left.

"Okay, Robert, the first thing we're going to do is go through your things and make sure that all of your belongings conform to our rules." He took my small bag, rifled through it, and told me I was good.

"Next, we're going to take your vitals," he said. So they took my blood pressure, pulse, and temperature.

"I'll walk you to your room," Tim said. "It's almost time for lunch. We're having grilled cheese sandwiches and tomato soup today."

I didn't much care about the lunch menu. I was disappointed that I wouldn't be getting any Librium.

We reached my room. Four beds made for a tight fit, and there wasn't much room to move around. I threw my bag on my bed and followed Tim to the cafeteria, which was a dingy room with a lot of disgusting people that I didn't want to be around. I went to the counter, got my lunch and a carton of milk, then sat at an empty table. My aim was to make it out of this place without having a seizure, getting beaten up, or having to interact with any lowlifes.

Each night after dinner, we would meet in the courtyard for an A.A. meeting. People from the outside would show up to run the meetings. Although I was never a fan of A.A., the meetings helped pass the time.

I learned from one of my roommates that several patients would scale the wall and get alcohol at a nearby Circle K. I also heard that other patients had friends throw drugs over the wall—mostly coke and meth. I hated that place, but I went through the motions until Friday, March 24, just after 5:00 p.m., when my sentence ended, and Ray came to fetch me.

He had some good news. He didn't think that I was mentally tough enough to stay in a shelter, and he was right. So, he managed to convince Therese to let me spend the weekend at their home, and on Monday, March 27, I would attend an interview that Ray had arranged at some no-frills halfway house called The Bootstrap Lodge. *Yippee ki-yay.*

CHAPTER 30

The Bootstrap Lodge

The weekend at Ray's was uneventful. I apologized to Brad for his having to see me carted off on a stretcher and into an ambulance. I also apologized to Therese, again, and thanked her for letting me spend the weekend with the family instead of at a shelter.

For the rest of the time, I pretty much kept to myself in my former bedroom. I read the newspaper and watched TV. I ate breakfast alone but had lunch and dinner with the family. I hadn't had a drink in ten days, and it was difficult watching Ray and Therese drink their beer and wine at mealtime.

Monday morning, Ray dropped me off at The Bootstrap Lodge, which was located just west of Campbell and a few blocks north of Grant Road.

As I got out of Ray's truck, he said to me, "Good luck. Call me when you find out if they're gonna let you in or not."

"Thanks," I said, "I'll let you know."

Ray drove off, and I walked toward the office. The door was wide open, and three men were gathered around a heavy-duty, gray-steel teacher's desk, laughing among themselves. The oldest of the three, who was probably in his late forties, and who I assumed was the boss, was seated in a chair behind the desk. The other two were sitting in beat-up wicker chairs. I tapped on the door.

"You must be Robert. What are you waiting for, an invitation?" asked the guy behind the desk. He seemed annoyed.

"We don't bite," said a younger guy, about thirty, sporting a cowboy hat and a bushy, straw-colored mustache. He spoke with a Texas twang.

The third guy, who was probably in his mid-thirties, didn't say anything. He appeared to be sizing me up.

I introduced myself and learned their names—the one seated at the desk chair was Ben, and he was indeed the director of the place. He was about six feet tall and wiry; he probably weighed about 170. He had a five o'clock shadow at 8:30 in the morning and salt and pepper gray hair that might have looked okay if not for his hack job of a haircut. Ben would turn out to be a megalomaniacal fucking bastard who treated everybody like shit and whose speech was laced with profanity.

Phil was the number two guy, and he was soft-spoken and humorless. He was tall, about 6'2, skinny, and pale. Shane was the Texan wanna-be, and he liked to talk. He was short but sturdily built.

Ben fixed his eyes on me and asked, "So, you want to live here? Tell us about yourself, and keep it short."

"Well," I said, "I'm easy to get along with, and I'm a hard worker."

"And . . . ?" Ben asked.

I tried to follow his lead and said, "And I don't want to drink anymore."

"Bingo," Ben said. "What about you two? Do you think he means what he says?"

Shane spoke up. "I don't know. Can you resist the lure of the golden triangle?" he asked me.

What the fuck kind of shit is this? I wanted to ask, but I needed to be respectful. "I'm afraid I don't know what the golden triangle is," I said. "Is it anything like the Bermuda Triangle?"

"Holy fuck, are you for fucking real?" Ben asked me. "The Bermuda fucking Triangle? Are you drunk right now?"

Phil and Shane laughed. I didn't like the way they were fucking with me.

"I give up," I said, trying to mask my anger. "What is the golden triangle, and why should I care?"

"Oh, the man's got some spunk after all," Phil said.

"Yeah," Ben said. "But he'd better not get too spunky. We're here to learn, not to bump heads."

I wasn't bumping anyone's fucking head. I did not like Ben one fucking bit, but I had to play along. I had nowhere else to go.

"Okay," Shane said to me. "You see the black box on the bookshelf behind you?"

I turned and spotted a black-framed shadow box, which was a twelve-by-twelve picture frame with a black door mounted on hinges. The backing was a light-colored matte. Secured to the matte was a shiny, gold-lamé-covered, three-dimensional, triangular pyramid. The triangle was probably ten by ten. It was tacky and garish.

"Okay," I said. "That's quite the conversation piece." I had the notion that it was somehow supposed to represent a woman's vagina.

"It's more than a conversation piece," Ben said. "It's educational and instructive. The golden triangle has been the downfall of many a good man. Are you catching my drift?"

I certainly was, so I said, "I'm guessing it represents a woman's genitalia, her vagina."

Ben laughed out loud. "What are you, some sort of faggot? It's not genitalia. It's not a vagina. It's a fucking pussy, and it represents all women."

Shane spoke, "It's a fucking statement that all women are trouble, and they will ruin your life with their golden, fucking triangles. Every pussy is dangerous. The Bootstrap Lodge is Dead Pecker Row, and we don't hunt beaver here."

I didn't say a word, but Ben said, "If you want to stay sober, to live here, you have to stay clear of the cunts."

"You're not a bad-looking guy," Phil said. "You're gonna run into women at A.A. meetings, and they're going to tempt you. Lead you astray. Are you prepared for that? Can you protect yourself from the golden triangle? If you can't commit to avoiding the golden triangle, you might as well march right out the door and pull up a stool at the nearest saloon."

"Well, sobriety will be my number one priority."

"My number one priority—quit shoveling the fucking shit," Ben said. "Will you stay away from the golden triangle or not? It's a simple fucking question."

I wanted to tell these assholes to go fuck themselves, but I was in a fix. I hoped that I could live there, get a job, and stay as far away from these three knuckleheads as possible.

Finally, I gave in. "Yes," I said, "I can avoid the golden triangle."

Ben stood up. "Well, color me green and call me Kermit. Gentlemen, I think Robert here is starting to get it."

"So," I asked, "does that mean I'm in?"

Ben said, "Yeah, you're in. But we have to go over some rules. First thing is, you have to find a job within one week. We're not a fucking charity. Next, we charge eighty-five bucks a week. The Bootstrap Lodge has some wealthy board members, so you can move in today and pay us what you owe once you're collecting a paycheck. But we aren't gonna let you sit on your ass. Ain't no handouts. You find a job, or you hit the road."

Phil continued, "We're almost at full capacity, so you're going to be living in a room with seven other guys. It has one bathroom and a shower. So, you'll hafta learn to get along and be patient."

Eight fucking guys and one bathroom, I thought. *That's fucking ridiculous.*

"We have thirty residents, including the three of us and a cook," Shane said. "Ben has his own room, and so does the cook. Phil and I share a room. Everyone else—well, we put 'em where we can fit 'em. You get three hots and a cot, and everybody but us and the cook takes a turn doing dinner dishes. Jesse, the cook, puts out cold cereal and milk for breakfast, and he makes biscuits and gravy, too. And there's a large coffee urn that's only available on weekday mornings. Jesse will give you a bagged lunch with a sandwich and chips, but ya gotta put your name on a list. Some guys who can afford it buy their lunch."

Phil spoke again, "And the rule about drinking is etched in stone—one strike and you're out. No second chances."

"You got all that?" Ben asked me.

"Yeah," I said, "I got it. Sounds fair enough."

"Shane will show you around," Ben said. "Most of the guys are at work, but you can see your bed and a drawer to keep your things in. And you better not waste time in the bathroom. No jackin' off either."

Shane and I walked to my new room. I couldn't believe it. There were four beds in one room, and two rooms had two beds each, but no doors. I got the only bed left, which was right next to the fucking bathroom. *What a fucking dump*, I thought. Shane then showed me a patio area with a bench and some free weights. It reminded me of Serenity Springs. I would spend a lot of time there and make some good friends. Shane walked with me to the cafeteria and the living room, which had a large couch, some beat-up old easy chairs, and a television.

I called Ray and told him that I'd been accepted. He sounded glad to be rid of me. The next morning, I was given money to take the bus to an employment agency. They had a job for me at a warehouse that packaged cheap, made-in-China stickers, pencils, and stationery for little girls. My hours were 5:30 a.m. to 4:00 p.m, with a half-hour lunch. The ten-hour days were mandatory, as were four hours every Saturday morning. The hours sucked, but I preferred being at work to hanging out at the Lodge. The pay was five bucks an hour, but with 14 hours a week overtime, I was grossing $305 a week, which made it easy to pay my back and current rent with a good deal left over. Ray and Therese gave me the orange bike, and that's how I got to and from work.

I met some decent guys, but no one who lived there had earned his charm school diploma. Most of them worked as roofers or carpenters. The place wasn't a haven for doctors and lawyers. Still, I had a roof over my head and three healthy meals each day. I had been through far worse.

We had to attend three A.A. meetings a week—all held at the Lodge. We met on Sundays, Wednesdays, and Fridays at 7:00, and once in a while, we'd have visitors, but it came as no surprise that hardly any women ever showed up.

As it turned out, Ben would wind up getting drunk and kicked out after I'd only been there about a month. I was glad to see him go. Phil took over as director, but he didn't cope well under pressure, and he wasn't good at giving orders. He also succumbed to the sauce and was given his walking papers. Next up was Shane. Shane was a natural. He was a born talker, and he reveled in being the head honcho. Shane even introduced a policy that whenever anybody got busted for drinking or using—and that happened a lot—"Another One Bites the Dust" by Queen would blare from a loudspeaker. The job turned him into even more of a dick than he was the day I met him.

After a few months, I got sick of the warehouse, so I quit. A guy at the house was working for a landscaping outfit, and he got me a job doing landscape construction. I dug a lot of trenches, planted a lot of trees, shrubs, and cactus, and learned how to install irrigation systems. It was hard work, but it kept me in shape. I was working ten-hour days and taking home over $300 a week, and I didn't have to work Saturdays. Life at The Bootstrap Lodge wasn't that bad if you were a skillful navigator.

I stuck it out at the Lodge until early June of 1996, when I moved into an apartment on the east side of town. By that time, I was driving a Yellow Cab and earning a decent living. But how would I fare without the rigid structure of the Lodge?

CHAPTER 31

Casa de Serenidad

After living at The Bootstrap Lodge for 15 months, I moved into a nice studio apartment near Pima and Craycroft on June 2. I spent that day driving a cab until 3:00 p.m., when I moved my few possessions into my new abode. Before turning in the cab at the end of my shift, I bought two cases of beer and two fifths of vodka, which I delivered to my new place. That June and early July, the average temperature was 102°, and the overnight temperature rarely dipped below 80°. On June 5, the air conditioning in my second-floor unit broke down. I was on day four of a full-blown binge. The heat in my apartment was stifling, but I was way too drunk to tell the apartment manager about the air conditioner breaking down.

I was spending all of my money on booze and some soup that I would drink cold, straight out of the can. I wasn't working, and my money was going fast. The rent for this unfurnished studio—and by unfurnished, I mean there was not a stick of furniture—was $350.00 a month and was due next on July 5. By the last week of June, I had about $50.00 to my name, and I was using a rolled-up sweatshirt for a pillow. I had a phone, which I never answered, and I had an answering machine. My friends from A.A. kept calling. Constantly. But I just wanted to be left alone.

Each morning, right before 6:00, when the Circle K opened its coolers, I would drink my last two beers and walk more than a mile to the store to buy an 18-pack of their cheapest brew. When I made it back to my apartment, I'd slam down three beers.

On Monday, July 1, I experienced what I knew was either pancreatitis or alcoholic gastritis, both of which I had been through several times before. I knew that neither would go away on its own. I'd have to visit the ER.

I managed to walk about two miles to the nearest hospital, the Pima County Medical Center. I was diagnosed with gastritis, which was less serious than pancreatitis. The ER crew was not sympathetic to my plight. It was clear that they viewed alcoholics as a waste of their time and energy, and who was I to disagree?

Nevertheless, my visit was not in vain. The doctors sent me home after giving me a shot of morphine. They just wanted to be rid of me. I also received some much-appreciated prescriptions that included Demerol for pain, Valium for alcohol withdrawal, and Compazine suppositories for nausea. I stopped at the Osco on my way home and filled my prescriptions.

I returned to my apartment and tore into the drugstore bags. I was too nauseated to hold anything down, not even a pill or a sip of water, so I unwrapped a suppository, wet it lightly with warm water, dropped my drawers, and inserted the magic bullet. Within about 20 minutes, the nausea had subsided, and I was enjoying a nice buzz from the sedative effects of the Compazine.

I still had a fifth of cheap vodka. I drank about six ounces from a glass and washed it down with tepid water from the kitchen tap. Then, I took a Valium, let it dissolve under my tongue, and fell asleep on the floor.

The following morning, I awoke extremely nauseated, so I inserted another Compazine suppository. In a matter of minutes,

I was feeling fine and enjoying my vodka again. I still hadn't taken any of the Demerol. I had a plan, and I would need it later. All of it.

On July 3, I had finished my vodka, so I walked to the Circle K at 6:00 a.m. and bought two twelve packs of Old Milwaukee Ice. I returned to my apartment and downed three cans of beer.

The ER doctor had prescribed 12 Compazine suppositories, 25 milligrams; 30 Demerol tablets, 100 milligrams; and 30 Valiums, blue, my favorite color, 10 milligrams each. By 1996, I had already been to several long-term alcohol rehabs, and the prospect of another was out of the question. I just wanted to fall asleep and never wake up. So, on that July 3 morning, with 21 beers remaining, I considered whether I had enough drugs and alcohol to go to sleep for keeps. It was time to find out.

I'd already used two Compazine suppositories, which left me ten. I planned to insert a Compazine missile every 30 minutes and drink four beers an hour. For me, fifteen minutes was plenty of time to polish off 12 ounces.

I estimated that it would take me five hours to finish both the Compazine and the beer. Near the end of that time, I would take the 30 Demerol tablets I had saved and the 27 Valiums I had left.

At 11:30 a.m., I put the Valiums into my mouth and washed them down with tap water. Next, I ingested the Demerol.

I drifted in and out of sleep most of that morning, but I stuck to my drinking schedule. At about noon, I fell into a deep sleep. It was a slumber that bordered on comatose. I awoke to a loud pounding on my door.

"Mr. Rickelman, are you inside? It's the police. We need you to open the door."

The pounding grew louder. I opened my eyes and tried to stand, but I was too drunk and heavily drugged.

Boom! Boom! Boom!

I thought the door would burst.

"Sir, please open the door. We are conducting a welfare check. We need to know that you are all right. Open the door immediately!"

Well, I didn't open the door, but the police did, with the help of the landlady. I was taken by ambulance to the Kino Community Health Center on East Ajo Way. I was out cold, but the ER staff inserted a nasogastric tube into my gut to administer charcoal and neutralize the lethal combination of booze and pills I'd consumed. I was then intubated and remained on a ventilator for two days.

Once I was stabilized, I was sent to the hospital's psych ward. This was the first time I'd ever been in a psych ward, and I was scared. The other patients told me that I should consider myself lucky. I was in the hospital's relatively peaceful West Ward, where the patients were generally cooperative, if not wholly lucid.

"Don't act up," came a warning from the regulars, "or they'll send you East, and you do not want to go East."

The nurses and psych techs confirmed that most of the patients in East Ward were hostile, belligerent, and oftentimes, violent.

I behaved myself and was always cooperative with the doctors and nurses. During my month-long stay, the doctors designated me as SMI, for Seriously Mentally Ill. After thirty years, I still carry that SMI designation.

The first few days in the psych ward weren't too bad. I received lots of Librium, two 25-milligram capsules every four hours, and chloral hydrate to help me sleep. I loved my meds, especially the chloral hydrate, that beautiful green gel cap that knocked me on my ass. I would take two, go to bed, and fall asleep in no time. I'd awaken like clockwork at 3:00 a.m. and request more Librium and chloral hydrate from the night nurse. I'd take my meds, return to my room, and fall fast asleep.

After five days, the Librium had done its job. The doctors replaced it with Ativan, which was not nearly as strong. Its calming effect wore off much more quickly than Librium's. Because the half-life of Ativan was shorter than Librium's, the doctors allowed me to ask for and receive it whenever I needed. That is referred to as "PRN," which in Latin means "pro re nata," or, loosely translated, "as the occasion arises." All the nurses were very compassionate, and since I wasn't asking too often, they always gave me my Ativan when I requested it. Until, that was, I met the nurse from hell. She was a matronly woman in her mid-fifties and was probably one of the last nurses on the planet who still wore the severe, starched uniform, complete with white shoes and stockings and, of course, the quintessential white nurse's cap. I guessed she liked the military effect, which said, "*I'm in charge. Do not fuck with me.*" In my shaky condition, I was in no mood to fuck with anyone. I just wanted to get through my ordeal with as little drama as possible.

For some reason, this nurse, who worked the evening shift, thought I was abusing the Ativan. Every time I asked for it, she would insist that I didn't need it. And I would very politely remind her that the doctor's orders were specific—PRN. She eventually gave in, until one night when she flat-out refused my request. I complained to one of the psych techs, and when Nurse Ratched learned of my complaint, she lost it. In a very loud voice, she summoned me to the nurses' station and, treating me like a fucking dog, said, "Come here, boy. C'mon, boy, come get your little white pill." I was mortified and incensed by her cruel behavior. Trembling like a leaf, I took a cup with the pill and downed it with a sip of water. My hands were shaking so badly that most of the water splashed on my shirt. I mustered the courage to mutter, "You're a horrible, old hag, and you shouldn't be a nurse."

Her face grew crimson against her white uniform. She said,

"You're nothing but a drunk who's trying every trick in the book to get as many drugs as you can. I see your type all the time."

"Well, I'm going to file a grievance against you," I said.

"Be my guest. Whose word is going to matter, mine or yours? Can you tell me that? Yes, you just be my guest."

The next day, I filed a grievance, and she never repeated that humiliating behavior. But I always dreaded approaching her for my PRNs. I spent much of my time devising plans to kill her when I got out. For some reason, I forgot to mention that to the doctors.

After my month-long stint, I left Kino and was put under the charge of a behavioral health service known as AYUDA, which operated several "step-down" units that were places for patients to live between their stays at psychiatric hospitals and subsequent stints at halfway houses. This place, called Casa de Serenidad, was a former apartment complex that was in surprisingly good condition. There were probably 50 to 60 units. I was in a four-bedroom apartment and had my own bedroom. When I moved in, I had two roommates, and one bedroom was vacant. Casa de Serenidad was a misnomer if ever there was one. There were many psychotic "tenants," and outbursts and altercations were commonplace. When I first got there, the place spooked me, but you get used to things, and I got used to—sort of—my whacked-out neighbors.

As far as roommates go, I was fortunate. There was Bob, who was bipolar, but his medications worked well, and he was easygoing and levelheaded. I considered him normal, but that is not a term favored by therapists or psychiatrists. I don't agree. I believe that there are parameters of normalcy, and "normal" people act within those parameters. "Abnormal" people do not. Where did I fit? Somewhere in between, I guessed.

Anyway, Bob was a fairly lucid guy who relied on a two-wheel walker to get around. He received an SSDI, or Social Security

Disability Insurance, check on the third of each month. By the financial standards at Serenidad, he was getting along quite well.

My other roommate, whose bedroom was directly across from mine, was Rick. Rick, unlike Bob, was not "fairly lucid." He was a pleasant, but full-blown, schizophrenic, who believed that major corporations had replaced our world's governments, and the game of *Rollerball* was being used to manipulate people in a manner not unlike the gladiator contests of ancient Rome. Rick was convinced that the United States was solidly under the control of corporate America, specifically, a cabal of Rollerball team owners. If this theory seems familiar, you may be remembering the plot of the 1975 movie, *Rollerball,* which featured James Caan as a star of the game. He represented the power of good and fought on the side of personal freedom to undermine the evil enterprises.

Sadly, in Rick's mind, the James Caan character did not exist, and most of us were in a bit of a pickle. But all was not lost. Rick had been hearing voices, transmissions rather, from an outer space visitor, a friendly one, who was willing to help battle the corporate villains. And there was more good news. This space alien, whose name Rick couldn't recall, had no designs on invading or conquering Earth. He only wanted to help us.

As Rick and Bob did not share the same mental illness, they were very different in appearance as well. Bob, who was probably in his mid-forties, was short, about 5'6, and going bald. And although he was thin, he had a considerable paunch.

Rick, on the other hand, was tall, probably 6'3, and although I never saw him do so much as one push-up, he was quite muscular, just one of those lucky, naturally well built guys. He was also younger than Bob, probably in his mid-twenties.

Rick was also receiving a monthly Social Security Disability check, and his sections of the refrigerator and cupboards were always well stocked with goodies. Rick had a loving and devoted father. It must have been heartbreaking for him to have a son whom he loved so much, but knew would never be "right." Rick's dad visited a few times a week and always brought something tasty for him to eat. And he brought coffee; Rick loved his coffee.

For those unfortunate ones, including me, who had no monthly check, there was the dining room. The food wasn't too bad, but you had to put up with several ranting, raving, and hysterical patients. I would always arrive just before the kitchen closed, and when the place was nearly empty. I avoided the other tenants whenever I could.

Rooms at Casa de Serenidad didn't stay vacant for long, and after five days, we had our fourth roommate. Gabe was a heavyset, young Hispanic man who was about 5'5 tops—and probably tipped the scales at 230. He had a nice head of shoulder-length, thick black hair. His healthy mane was starkly contrasted by his baby face. Gabe had no facial hair whatsoever.

He, too, was a lucky recipient of the SSDI check.

Within two days of moving in, Gabe developed the habit of bringing home a bag of Nacho Cheese Doritos, some extra-long Slim Jims, and a six-pack of 16-ounce Budweisers. Some days, I would consider turning him in for the drinking, but he was pretty laid back, and I figured we could have wound up with a much worse roommate. So, Gabe stayed, drinking his Budweisers and enjoying his Slim Jims and Doritos until his luck ran out early one evening when he came home totally shit-faced. He was gone the same night.

One nice thing about Serenidad was that my nighttime regimen of chloral hydrate and Ativan was continued, both the bedtime and the 3:00 a.m. doses. Then things changed. One very early morning of my third week, I awoke for my 3:00 a.m. dose and was informed by a snarky night nurse that this would be my last early morning dose of chloral hydrate. The following week, it would be DC'd, that is, discontinued altogether. I was stunned and indignant.

"Do you think it's funny that my meds are being DC'd?" I asked.

She smirked and informed me, "The DC is per your doctor's orders."

"I have a doctor? What are you talking about? I've been here for three weeks and I've never seen a doctor."

"His name is Dr. Patterson, and he's very busy. You're not his only client. Have you looked around this place?"

"Can I talk to him?" I asked.

"You can try. Like I said, he's a busy man."

"Well," I said, "just so you know, I think you are a heartless bitch who has no soul."

"Enjoy your meds, Robert. He who laughs last; know what I mean?"

She had me. All I could manage was a tired, "Fuck you."

I walked slowly back to bed to savor my chloral hydrate. I spent most of that week trying to get an appointment with Dr. Patterson.

"He'll see you when his schedule allows," was the common refrain.

The days passed, and I took my final dose of chloral hydrate, rushing to bed to enjoy its full effects. At least I still had my Ativan. But instead of getting one milligram every four hours, I received it every six. From the moment I swallowed it, I waited for my next dose.

Then, one morning at 11:40, I lay in bed waiting for my noon dose. There was an unexpected knock on my bedroom door. I was puzzled, and a little unnerved. Nobody knew where I was, so I was not expecting any visitors. I opened the door. Standing in the threshold was a man whom I took to be a doctor, accompanied by two burly psych techs.

"Hello, Robert, I'm Doctor Patterson. I understand that you've been asking to see me."

Finally, I thought, *I can talk some sense into this doctor, and get my chloral hydrate back.*

"Yes, Doctor, I wanted to know why my chloral hydrate has been DC'd, and why my Ativan dose was lowered," I said.

He rubbed his brow with his left hand. "I'm sorry, Robert, but I believe that you were on the chloral hydrate for far too long, and at much too high a dose. And as far as the Ativan is concerned, that too is being discontinued. You won't be receiving any more, effective immediately."

"But . . . when . . . I have my noon dose in 20 minutes. I am going to get that, right?"

"I'm sorry, Robert, but you won't be receiving any more Ativan."

"But that's not fair. I've been waiting, expecting my noon dose. I need my Ativan."

"That's why we're going to keep you here for the next few weeks to make sure that there are no complications from taking you off these meds. You need to be clean before you can move on. And we plan on moving you to a facility with more highly functioning clients. I think that will work well for you."

I was silent, stunned.

"You see, Robert, you're being placed in a halfway house for men who, like you, have been dually diagnosed, which means that not only are you suffering from a mental illness, but you're addicted to a substance, any substance. In your case, alcohol. The place is called Safe Harbor. Like Serenidad, it's a former apartment complex, but much nicer and, more importantly, much more serene. I've been there. It's clean, quiet, and the atmosphere is very relaxed. Especially compared to the little cuckoo's nest we're running here." He allowed himself a half-smile.

"But," he said, "they don't allow their clients to take controlled substances, and that's why we're discontinuing your Ativan. By the way, the chloral hydrate that you were so fond of is also a controlled substance."

I shrugged with an air of quiet resignation.

"Believe me, Robert, this is a good move for you. We're going to try to find a medication that fits the criterion of no benzodiazepines, but addresses what I see as very severe anxiety and depression."

"How am I supposed to sleep? First, the chloral hydrate, which was bad enough, now the Ativan?"

"Tonight, we'll be giving you Benadryl to help you sleep."

"Benadryl? Are you serious?"

"Benadryl can be a very effective sleep agent," he said.

"What if it doesn't work?"

"Then, Robert, we have a variety of drugs that can help you sleep. I'll be seeing you daily while you're here. We'll find an effective medication for the symptoms that you're presenting. I'll see you in my office tomorrow morning at 10:00. Just try to relax. We're here to help you."

I was dismayed, but he was the doctor. I received the Benadryl that night, and it didn't do shit. The following morning, at 10:00, I was seated in Dr. Patterson's office.

"Robert, I've been looking at your files from here and from Kino. Clearly, you're suffering from severe depression, as well as generalized anxiety disorder. We're going to address your anxiety and depression with two medications, which don't conflict with the controlled substance restrictions at Safe Harbor. The first is Zoloft. We'll start you on 50 milligrams daily for a week and see if we should increase the dose or possibly try a different medication. My thought is that we'll bring you up to 100 milligrams, and if you feel no relief or experience any discomfort, we'll prescribe a different medication.

"Now, as for sleep, there is an antidepressant that's been around for several years. It's called Trazodone. This drug has a side effect that should prove beneficial to you. You see, in the great majority of patients, Trazodone produces very pronounced drowsiness. So, in light of your problem sleeping, I'm going to put you on 150 milligrams to take at bedtime, and if that doesn't do the trick, we'll raise it to 300. How does that sound?"

I smiled. "Thank you so much, Doctor. That sounds great. It's so nice to finally have a plan and to understand what's happening with me."

"I see you attended the University of Illinois and spent three semesters in law school," he said. "I am pleased when the patient understands what he is taking and why. By all means, don't hesitate to ask questions. I also see that your father was an attorney and that he had issues with your dropping out of law school."

"He thinks I'm a loser."

"Well, Robert, I don't think that you are by any means a loser. And we're going to connect you with a therapist to work on this and other issues as you move on."

I couldn't believe my luck. Funny, my first impression of Dr. Patterson was that he was a pompous asshole. Now, I saw him in a completely different light. Maybe, after so many wasted years, I was going to get my life on track.

After a week, the 150 milligrams of Trazodone weren't doing the trick, so as promised, the doctor raised the dose to

300 milligrams. Finally, I was able to sleep through the night. Regrettably, I was getting no benefit from the Zoloft. The doctor raised the dose to 100 milligrams to see if the increase would improve my mood and anxiety.

"We'll give the Zoloft another week, and if you don't feel any improvement, we'll discontinue it and try something else. There are several medications that address anxiety and depression. Sometimes it's just hit and miss."

"Hit and miss," I said.

"I'm sorry, Robert, but there is so much about our brains that we're just beginning to learn, and, right now, there's no wonder drug. But with you and me working together, I promise, in time, we will find the answer you're looking for. That you deserve."

Finally, in early September of 1996, the day came for me to move into Safe Harbor. I was pretty nervous about the whole thing. I now had a case manager to help me navigate the behavioral health system. Her name was Carol Prentice, and she was very nice. She'd been sober for over ten years. I had never known anyone with ten years of sobriety.

The Safe Harbor clients—all men—were housed in a separate area in the rear of an apartment complex called Nueva Esperanza, which served strictly as a rehab for addicts and alcoholics. It housed both men and women. None of those clients had been diagnosed with mental disorders. As a rule, we didn't mix with the others. It might have been my paranoia, but they seemed to think that they were better than us. We were the crazy guys. I didn't mind our being kept apart. As for the female clients, most of them were pretty rough trade. Once in a while, there'd be a cute young girl, but those guys at Nueva Esperanza were always sniffing for a piece of ass. I was already 41 years old and considered myself over the hill. I left the women alone.

Every Safe Harbor client was required to do volunteer work. I was taking Nardil, an antidepressant, and I was doing well. I began working for an agency that provided services for the visually impaired. That's where I met Pat, who was hired as a social worker at the agency in August of 1997. She was gorgeous, and I developed an instant crush on her. I considered her way out of my league, but for some inexplicable reason, Pat had feelings for me, too. We started dating in the spring of 1998, and that September, we were married.

My poor Pat—she met me when the Nardil was working. Things were great until it gradually lost its effect; the doctors began experimenting with a series of other drugs. I tried more than 20 psychotropic meds, and that turned my life and Pat's completely upside down. She hadn't signed on for the misery and heartache I put her through, but she stayed with me, and I will always love her for that.

CHAPTER 32

Psychokinesis

It was a Tuesday night in early March. Pat had obtained a court order for me to spend 72 hours on a psych hold. According to the order, I was a danger to myself. This wasn't the first time I'd been held for psychiatric observation. I didn't want to be in this hospital, but I knew it was for my own good and that Pat needed a break from my self-destructive behavior.

I walked into the recreation room and was glad to find it empty. The movie *Armageddon* was playing, and I sat down to watch. That's when a young woman entered and took a seat in one of the worn-out leather recliners.

"Hi, I'm Aimee," she said. "Can I ask you a question?"

"Hi, Aimee. I'm Rob. Sure, ask me whatever you'd like."

This woman was sending out some peculiar vibes. She wasn't your run-of-the-mill psych patient. We all have a certain weirdness quotient; I know that. But with her, I felt strangely defenseless and vaguely in peril. From what, I couldn't say, but the danger was palpable.

She stood and faced me. "Look at me," she said. "Do I have camel toe?"

Camel toe. Jeez. That's a very graphic reference to a woman's pants riding up her crotch and drawing attention to where your eyes shouldn't be looking.

"Camel toe? No . . . no, I didn't notice."

"Well, take a closer look. Do I?"

A closer look—what the fuck . . . I obliged her, quickly scanning the area in question. She was very pretty—petite, about five foot two, maybe 110 pounds. Her skin was golden and smooth, her brown eyes sparkled, and her full, round lips were a soft pink. She had sleek black hair that was cut short, and her thick round bangs just reached her eyebrows.

"No," I finally answered. "No, you don't."

"Thank you for checking."

What was I supposed to say? *My pleasure*?

"You're married, aren't you?" she asked. I wasn't wearing my wedding band. I think the intake people were afraid I'd swallow it.

"Good guess; yes, I am married."

"It wasn't a guess. I'm psychic. I can tell you the name of your wife."

"Okay, what's my wife's name?"

"It's coming to me. Kelli. Your wife's name is Kelli."

"Sorry, it's Pat."

"Okay, but I will tell you this—your Karma's in serendipity."

I had no inkling of what that meant.

"So, what can you do?" I asked.

"Well, I'm psychokinetic. I can move things using only my mind."

"That sounds cool. Can you move something in here?"

"Like what?"

We were in the TV room, so I suggested the DVD player.

"Get ready; here goes."

I wasn't surprised when nothing happened.

Not missing a beat, she declared, "You know, I can blow up a light bulb just by willing it to explode. I mean *implode* it—I don't want to hurt anyone."

Gesturing to the ceiling, I asked, "Can you implode one of these fluorescent lights?"

"Hmmm . . . fluorescent's a lot harder than regular light bulbs. But, I'll tell you what, tomorrow at breakfast, I'll implode every light in the cafeteria. Everyone's going to freak out!"

"I'm looking forward to that," I said. "You know, the last time I was here, I met a woman who said she was a medium."

"A medium, right. What'd she do? Never mind, it doesn't matter. I don't believe in that medium crap. Mediums claim they can communicate with the dead. I don't believe in ghosts and all that spooky mumbo jumbo."

I didn't say anything. I just sort of shuffled my feet.

"Do I make you nervous?" she asked.

"A little."

"I can tell. You're cute when you're nervous. You're a genius, aren't you? The reason I know is that I'm a genius too."

"Genius?" I asked. "I don't really think I'm a genius."

"I wasn't always a genius myself, but the strangest thing happened to me after I was hit by a car. I wasn't hurt bad, but—and this is amazing—after the accident, my intelligence went sky high. And, ever since, I can speak 14 languages. French, Italian, Spanish, German, Chinese. You name it, I can speak it."

"Well," I said, "It's been a long day and I'm pretty tired. I guess I should say, '*Bonne nuit.*'"

"Excuse me?"

"Good night. I said good night in French."

"Oh, yeah. You kind of mumbled it."

"Sorry."

"Es tarde y estoy muy cansado. It's late, and I'm very tired," I

said.

"I don't need a translator. I told you I was fluent in—"

"Yes, 14 languages."

"Wait," she said. "Can I ask you a big favor?"

I wanted to get out of there, but I nodded. "Sure, then I have to get to bed so my sleep meds will work."

"Yeah, the window." She meant the window of opportunity that the sleep meds need to work. If you lose that window, you could be up all night.

"So, what can I do for you before I hit the sack?"

"Would you please kiss me? On the lips."

She didn't just ask me to kiss her; she couldn't have. Holy fucking shit.

"I'm sorry, Aimee. I'm very happily married."

"Just one kiss. I promise. Perfectly innocent."

"I can't. Really, I just can't."

"Do you think I'm pretty? I know you do."

"Aimee, I think you're beautiful, but . . . my wife. I can't kiss you. I love my wife."

"Okay, then just a quick kiss on my cheek."

"I'm sorry, I just ca—"

Before I knew it, she'd planted a soft kiss on my mouth. The kiss caught me off guard and left me bewildered and uneasy.

"How was that?" she asked.

"Very nice," I said. "That was a very nice kiss." I was blushing. I could feel the warmth on my face.

"G'night," she said. "I can't wait to blow out the lights in the morning. You're gonna love it."

"I'm looking forward to it. Good night, Aimee."

Feeling lightheaded and a bit guilty, I headed to the safety of my room.

The next morning, the cafeteria lights remained intact. There was not so much as a burned-out bulb. But something was off. I felt like every staff member was eyeing me judgmentally. Had someone seen "the kiss," and even if they had, how was that my fault?

CHAPTER 33

Antabuse

I sat in a chair in the office of the hospital psychiatrist, a darkly handsome man in his late thirties. His name was Dr. Mohammed Khatana, and I guessed from his accent that he was from Pakistan. He read my file carefully. I was still detoxing, and my entire body was trembling. I was taking 50 milligrams of Librium every six hours to help with the withdrawal. I couldn't imagine how terrible I would be feeling without the benzos.

"So," he said, as he looked up from his papers, "nine long-term alcohol rehabs, eleven psychiatric hospitals, petitioned once, chronic and acute pancreatitis, several bouts of alcoholic gastritis. And yet, you continue to drink. We have quite a dilemma on our hands, haven't we?"

I nodded in agreement.

"I'm sure the topic of using Antabuse must have been raised over so many years of treatment. But I don't see anything in your file to the effect that you have ever been prescribed this medication. Would you consider trying it? I feel that if we don't address this immediately, things are going to end badly for you."

"Well," I said, "I guess I've never wanted to take Antabuse because, deep down, I've always wanted to have the option of drinking if things got too bad. Also, my A.A. sponsor has told me that anyone who takes Antabuse is not truly sober, but I know he is wrong and that I'm just using his opinion as an excuse for not taking it. Besides, I think he's a bit of an asshole."

Dr. Khatana smiled. He'd probably never called anyone an asshole.

"Perhaps it's time to look for a new sponsor and to give yourself a fighting chance to stay sober."

"You know what, Doctor," I said, "I'm gonna quit with all the excuses, and I'm going to say yes to the Antabuse."

"I'm very pleased to hear that, Robert. We have to try to break this cycle of unsafe drinking and consequential hospitalizations. Let's say enough is enough. I'm going to have the hospital pharmacy start you on 250 milligrams per day, and I'm going to prescribe three months' worth of disulfiram, which is the generic form of Antabuse. You'll be taking 250 milligrams once a day for two weeks, then a maintenance dose of 500 milligrams, which you will also take once per day. The pharmacist will surely warn you, but I want to stress that drinking and taking Antabuse can be extremely dangerous. At the very least, it will make you severely ill, and it might even kill you. I cannot emphasize enough that you mustn't drink within forty-eight hours of taking it. And bear in mind that a severe reaction to alcohol may occur as long as two weeks after your last dose. Do you have any questions, Robert?"

"No, not really, Doctor. I've read up on Antabuse, and I know I'll have to stay away from anything containing alcohol, like mouthwash and cologne, which I don't use anyway. And I know to avoid things like wine vinegar, so none of that will be a problem."

"Very good, then. In a few months, your doctor will likely order labs such as liver function tests to make sure that your body is tolerating the medicine. Other than that, I believe you're good to go." He stood up and extended his hand. "Okay, so you will continue on the Librium, and you'll begin the Antabuse tomorrow. I truly believe that you can stay sober, and I wish you the very best."

I shook his hand. "Thank you, Doctor," I said. I left his office unsure of how committed I would be to taking my Antabuse. I was glad to be starting it while I was still in the hospital, where I would be for three more days. During that time, there were no side effects. On the afternoon of my discharge, I called Pat to pick me up, and the staff gave me a bag with my clothes as well as the discharge papers and a prescription for Antabuse. A psych tech escorted me to the patient pick-up area, where Pat was waiting. Her face reflected her apprehension. I couldn't blame her for worrying about taking me back home. I wasn't a good risk, but she was happy that I had agreed to take the Antabuse.

As Pat drove home, I reminded her that I had to drop off the prescription at the pharmacy. We went to the supermarket near our house, and I ran in while Pat waited in the car. I reached the pharmacy counter and was mortified to see that the clerk was an extremely attractive young woman. I handed her the prescription, feeling as if I had the word "DRUNK" stamped on my forehead. She glanced at the prescription and told me that it would be ready in twenty minutes.

"Thanks," I said. "I'll wait for it."

"Fine," she said.

I walked away feeling sheepish, but I doubt she gave our encounter a second thought.

I didn't have my phone, so I walked to the car to tell Pat that I was going to wait for the prescription to be filled. I just wanted to get the Antabuse and get the hell out of there. It was a pleasant late December afternoon, about sixty-five degrees. Pat said she would wait in the car, and I headed back into the store and took a seat near the pharmacy counter.

Within just a few minutes, I heard my name called.

I stood and said, "I'm Robert." It was the same pretty girl. *Rats,* I thought. *Just my luck. Why couldn't I get a fat old lady to fill this?*

But once again, the young woman was all business. Because I had the diagnosis of "Seriously Mentally Ill," there was no charge for the medicine.

"Our pharmacist would like to speak with you; answer any questions you might have," she said.

"Okay, I'd like his input," I said.

The pharmacist pretty much repeated what Doctor Khatana had told me, with a strong caveat of staying away from alcohol.

I thanked him, and I was out of there. As for the young woman, she could not have cared less what kind of prescription I had filled. And things could have been worse. At least I wasn't filling a prescription for Viagra. There was always a bright side if you just took a moment to look for it. I walked to the car, and Pat drove us home.

Well, I didn't give the Antabuse a fighting chance. At first, Pat would give me the tablet each morning, and I stayed off the sauce. But within a few weeks, I would cheek the pill that Pat gave me and spit it into my nearly empty cup of coffee when she turned away. After a few days, I was drinking again, and—soon—I was back to mixing my psych meds with booze. That was a very dumb decision.

CHAPTER 34

Danger to Self and Others

By mixing my meds with alcohol, I was soon a fucking mess. On February 3, 2003, I was petitioned and court-ordered for an involuntary psychiatric evaluation at Saint Mary's Hospital. While I was a patient there, the Pima County Attorney's office served me with a Notice of Hearing for Court-Ordered Treatment. I remained at the hospital until my hearing date before an Arizona Superior Court judge on Monday, February 24. The hearing room was located on a lower floor of the hospital.

According to Title 36 of the Arizona Revised Statutes, when you're petitioned, usually by a family member or a psychiatrist, you are remanded to a psychiatric hospital until a hearing is held to determine if, by reason of a mental disorder, you meet any of these four criteria: "[You are] a danger to yourself (DTS); a danger to others (DTO); persistently or acutely disabled (PAD); gravely disabled (GD)."

The process is intimidating. If things go badly, you can wind up at the Arizona State Hospital, or ASH, which is located in Phoenix. The stakes are high for a patient who is being evaluated by the judge.

The maximum periods of inpatient treatment that the court may order are as follows:

1. Ninety days for a person found to be a danger to himself.

2. One hundred eighty days for a person found to be a danger to others.

3. One hundred eighty days for a person found to have a persistent or acute disability.

4. Three hundred sixty-five days for a person found to have a grave disability.

The patients I saw leave our floor to attend their hearings didn't care much about how they were dressed. Most simply wore their hospital scrubs, or maybe a pair of sweatpants and a T-shirt. I, on the other hand, put a lot of effort into looking clean and well-dressed for my hearing before the judge. That morning, I was sporting a crisp pair of khaki slacks, a brand-new blue Oxford shirt that Pat had bought for me, and brown dress shoes (loafers, as hospital rules forbade shoes with laces). I asked the hospital staff if I could wear my new brown belt, but they would not allow it. Belts and shoelaces could be used to hang oneself, so they were prohibited.

Lawrence Kendrick, my court-appointed attorney, whom I'd met only once, for a ten-minute consult, was present. Pat, who was always in my corner, was there for moral support. My father and I had reconciled, and he and his future wife, Elise, were there as well.

Assessments had been prepared by two psychiatrists, both of whom determined that I was not only a danger to myself, but was a danger to others, persistently and acutely disabled, and gravely disabled. They'd checked all the boxes. The judge advised me that he was accepting the doctors' diagnoses that confirmed my designation of Seriously Mentally Ill. I'd been labeled SMI since 1996, so this was no surprise.

Although I was very nervous, I comported myself well, and when it was my turn to testify, I came off as lucid, coherent, and rational. The last thing I wanted was to end up at ASH, so I tried to persuade the judge that, although I had been a danger to myself, I was willing to enroll in a long-term rehab near my home.

The judge was amenable to my request and allowed me to live as a voluntary patient at the rehab I had chosen. If I finished 90 days without a problem, I would not be ordered to a long-term psych hospital. I thanked the judge and left the hearing with my lawyer. While I was thanking him in the lobby, he told me that I'd done a good job and asked if I had ever considered practicing law. I laughed and said no.

"Well, you should think about it," he said. "You presented a very well considered defense in there."

He shook my hand and left. Pat came and gave me a big hug. Then, my father and Elise each embraced me. I was going to be released that same day, and Pat would drive me to the rehab, a place called Las Lomas. I said goodbye and thank you to my dad and Elise, and gave my dad another hug. I wondered what he was thinking. I had shown so much promise in high school and college, and as far as he knew, during my first year of law school. But those were old promises, and they would never be fulfilled.

While Pat waited in the lobby, I found my friends in a group meeting and told them the good news. Lark, a young woman who preferred life on the streets, seemed especially happy for me. I said my goodbyes to the staff, gathered my belongings, and met Pat in the lobby. I felt uneasy as we drove to Las Lomas.

We reached my new residence, and Pat parked the car. A hard-looking woman, about fifty or so with bright red hair and a sturdy frame, met us at the car.

"Hi, you must be Robert," she said. "I'm Sheila."

I shook her hand. "Yes, I'm Robert. It's nice to meet you, Sheila. This is my wife, Pat."

"Hi," Pat said. "Well, I guess I'd better be going. Call me."

I kissed her on the cheek. "I will. Thank you so much for standing by me. I love you."

"I love you, too," she said as she walked to the car.

"Well, Robert, let's go inside, and we'll check to make sure that everything you brought is okay to keep," Sheila said.

We walked inside. I sat in an easy chair as she went through my things. I didn't have much, and I knew she wouldn't find any contraband.

"Looks like you're good," she said. I put my belongings back in my bag.

"Okay. I'll walk you to the house where our new residents stay for the first week. There's plenty of food, a TV, and some board games. After a week, you'll move into one of our apartments."

We walked to the house where I met the other three men who were living there. I soon learned that it served two levels of clientele. The house was the holding area for new patients and allowed the staff to gauge the level of mental illness of each newcomer. I was the only new patient living at the house. It was also long-term housing for hard-core, delusional men who needed twenty-four-hour supervision. They met the criteria for gravely disabled. One was a very large young man named Stanley. Stanley was about six feet tall and easily weighed over 300 pounds. Fortunately, for such a formidable man, Stanley was refreshingly good-natured.

"Stanley is our big eater around here," Sheila said.

I'd soon see for myself that he could consume more food than anyone I'd ever met. He ate so much that after dinner, staff would lock the cupboards and the refrigerator until breakfast. In the morning, Stanley would devour an entire box of cereal. The bowl he used was huge.

In addition to Stanley, there was Christian, an eighteen-year-old schizophrenic. Christian was strikingly handsome. He was tall, about six foot two, with long, unruly hair and slate-gray eyes. I'm sure that if he had not been so severely mentally ill, Christian might have been quite the ladies' man. But he kept mostly to himself. There were two mandatory meetings, one at 7:30 in the morning and the other at 6:00 in the evening. The guys in the house were not required to attend, but once in a while, Christian would show up for the evening meeting. He never made the morning meeting, as, every day, he slept well into the afternoon. At the evening meeting, we were supposed to sit in a circle and share how our days had gone. When Christian's turn came around, he would display an oddly serene smile and simply say, "Nothing happened today."

The other client who lived full-time in the house was an old man with a nasty temper. His name was Roger, and I steered clear of him.

We had a phone in our living room, which was nice because the only other one was in the recreation room. That phone would be a source of constant arguments over whose turn it was to use it, and accusations about clients monopolizing it.

As I was settling into our cozy living room to watch TV, a resident arrived asking for Robert. "That's me. I'm Robert," I said.

"Well, you have a phone call in the rec room. Some chick."

I rose from my comfy chair. "Thanks," I said. I walked to the rec room, hoping that Pat was calling.

The phone was on a small table near the door. I picked it up and said hello.

"Hi, Rob, guess who."

Shit, I thought. It was Lark. *Why was she calling me on my very first day at Las Lomas?*

"Hi, Lark. You didn't waste any time, did you? I haven't even settled in yet."

"Boy, I was expecting a heartier greeting than that. How are you, Rob? How do you like your new place?"

"Well, they've got me living in a small house with three other guys. They seem even crazier than me, but they're okay, and I only have to stay in the house for a week. Then I move into an apartment. I'm hoping to get my own place. I'll find out later. So, how are you?"

"Man, I'm getting real tired of this place, but my hearing date hasn't been set yet. I don't know what's taking them so long. I've been here for six fucking weeks now, and I know those assholes are going to send me to ASH anyway. But the reason I called was to ask for a huge favor."

My stomach clenched. I knew what was coming. "You know," I said, "I can't leave this place without supervision for a week. What did you need?"

"I could really use something to get high on. I'm sick of the lame doses of Ativan they give us. I would die to get my hands on some meth or something like that."

Meth. I knew it. I fucking knew she would ask me to get her some meth. What a selfish, fucking bitch. She didn't give two shits about my recovery or about my getting caught and kicked out of there.

"Wow, I don't know what to say. I don't know anybody who does meth or any of that shit. I just drink alcohol. I've never done meth. You know that."

"Yeah, but with all the guys living where you are, can't you find someone who can visit me and bring me something good?"

"No, Lark. I don't know anyone who could do that, and I'm not gonna risk getting kicked out of here. Not for you, not for anyone."

"Even after all the times I cheeked my Ativans for you? You're some kind of friend."

"Look," I said. "Pat and I bought you a lot of things you didn't have the money for. We bought you everything you asked for. I can't get you any drugs. Sorry."

There was a long pause, and then she said, "Man, I would have done it for you."

"Take care of yourself, Lark. I hope your hearing goes well and you can straighten out your life. That's what I'm trying to do here."

"Yeah, well, you do that. Thanks for nothing." She hung up, and I was relieved, but I was shaking like mad. I needed to stay clear of her and her schemes. She never called again, and I never called her. I don't know if she wound up at ASH or back on the streets. She was going to die out there, and there was nothing I could do about it. I hung up the phone and took some deep breaths. Then, I walked back to the house and went to my room to lie down. I fell into a very deep sleep and didn't wake up until 5:00 the next morning. That entire day had worn me out.

After a week of playing Scrabble and watching TV, mostly about when President Bush was going to invade Iraq, it was time to move into an apartment. I thanked my lucky stars that I was getting my own studio on the second floor. I received frequent visits from Sheila, who gave me my meds twice a day. The way it worked was that, once a week, Sheila would fill a small metal safe with all my daily medications. She would then lock the safe and keep the key. Every morning and evening, Sheila would come by to unlock my safe and give me my meds.

It was a very efficient policy, but it was not foolproof. One night, a patient suffering a psychotic episode broke into his safe and ingested all the medications that were in his box. Fortunately, when he stumbled out his door, a resident saw him, notified staff, and an ambulance was called. He was rushed to the hospital, where they pumped his stomach and saved his life.

After this incident, patients were scrutinized more closely for suicidal tendencies, and those who were judged as overdose risks were brought only enough medication for one dose.

At this time, I was taking 1 milligram of Ativan twice daily, as well as 400 milligrams of the mood stabilizer, Seroquel, and 75 milligrams of Effexor, which is an antidepressant. I'll say one thing about Ativan. It's better than nothing.

I would have preferred Klonopin, which I had been prescribed for several months in 2001, and which I found extraordinarily effective. I was taking 2mg of Klonopin three times daily, and my anxiety was reduced considerably. However, the doctors believed that it was not a safe medication, so they discontinued it. I suffered mightily from the withdrawal symptoms that attacked me when it was DC'd. As it turned out, for me, Klonopin was not the "drug from hell" that the young woman, Pilar, had warned me about when I was a patient some years earlier at ACHIEVE. In 2004, I was once again prescribed Klonopin, and I am still taking 2mg twice a day. It remains a vital component of my daily drug regimen.

Las Lomas was home to about thirty men, and there were some real characters. Christian from the house had a friend at Las Lomas, who, like him, was eighteen years old. His name was Alan; he was lazy, and he complained about everything. He lived in a two-bedroom apartment with Jeff, a very engaging individual who was quite the complainer in his own right. When I moved into my apartment, Jeff and Alan were my next-door neighbors. Alan had a huge stereo system that he played very loudly. I was constantly asking him to turn down the music. He would for a few minutes, but then he would crank the volume right back up. I appealed to Sheila to make Alan keep the noise down, but she had bigger fish to fry.

Another interesting character was Trevor. Trevor was twenty-one years old and was very much into rap music. He liked to call rapping "Spitting some bars." I liked that phrase. He was a good-looking kid and had a great sense of humor. Everyone liked to hang out with him. But he also had a dark side. Trevor was the patient who had busted open his drug box and taken all his meds. Sadly, he would not stay around long enough to "graduate" from Las Lomas. The siren song of crystal meth would wear down Trevor's defenses. He left, and I never learned what became of him. We had lost a bright, funny, good-hearted guy.

Alan's roommate, Jeff, was a cutter. His hands and arms were streaked with scars from razor blades and broken glass. He was constantly complaining to staff about petty issues, and he was always at odds with Alan over his loud music. But Jeff was an excellent storyteller. My favorite tale, which, based on Jeff's behavior at Las Lomas, I believe to be true, concerned an incident that took place at a halfway house where he had been living.

According to Jeff, he grew so fed up with his situation at the halfway house that, on an extremely cold night, he packed his few belongings and announced that he was moving out. This announcement was received gladly by the house manager. Jeff marched out and, after walking about a mile in the frigid night air, he decided that leaving had been a mistake. So Jeff picked up a large rock and smashed himself in the head. He struck himself with such force that he passed out and fell unconscious to the cold, hard ground.

When Jeff came to, he got up and headed back to the halfway house. He was bleeding badly and admitted to smashing his head with the rock; he pleaded to be readmitted. Fortunately for Jeff, the manager allowed him to return. But the story showed how readily inclined he was to hurt himself.

Then there was Aaron, who suffered from anxiety and panic attacks. When the group from Las Lomas was taken to the annual Tucson Rodeo Parade, Aaron, in the midst of a large crowd of parade watchers, clutched his chest and dropped to the ground, certain that he was suffering a heart attack. A fire department ambulance arrived, and Aaron admitted that he had misread his panic for a more serious condition. The paramedics decided that he was fine and left. Aaron would suffer many more panic attacks during his stay at Las Lomas.

While I was in the back of our big white van, returning from the parade, I got into a discussion with a patient named Brad, who suffered from bipolar depression and schizophrenia. I happened to mention that one of the side effects of anti-psychotics was tardive dyskinesia.

"Yeah," said Brad, "I take Haldol, and I have that tardive dyskinesia."

I looked at him closely. He was constantly smacking his lips and moving his eyebrows up and down. And his hands shook severely.

God, I thought, *I hope that never happens to me.*

"How long have you been taking Haldol?" I asked.

"Well, let's see. I was at ASH for seven years. I'm pretty sure they started the Haldol right after I got there. My memory's not so good anymore."

"You were at ASH for seven years? Damn."

"Yeah, like I said, my memory's not too good, but I know I was at a party. That part I remember. So, anyway, I was at this party, and I guess I got into an argument with two guys. And I stabbed them both with a knife. One of them almost died."

"Fuck," I said.

"Yeah, I was surprised when I woke up in jail and they told me what happened."

There was a flatness to his voice, no emotion. I think the psychiatrists call it a "blunted affect." That is an excellent description.

"So, you didn't go to prison?"

"No, Arizona has something called, umm . . ."

"Guilty Except Insane; Section 13-502." It was Aaron. He had recovered from his panic attack.

"Yeah, that's it, Guilty Except Insane," Brad said. "So I did seven years at ASH, which is probably how long I would have gone to prison. They could have kept me longer, but the doctors said I had improved and wasn't a danger to myself or others. It's all up to the doctors—the psychiatrists. When I got out, they sent me here."

"Wow. So, seven years at ASH. I guess that beats prison," I said.

"Sure does," said Aaron. "I tried to kill my girlfriend, and I got Guilty Except Insane and did five years at ASH."

"What if you do kill somebody?" I asked, astonished.

"The judge can use it even if you kill somebody. But, if the shrinks don't think you're getting better, they can keep you a whole lot longer than the time you would have spent in prison."

"Were you guys drunk when you did that stuff?" I asked.

"No," Aaron said. "If you're drunk or high, you can't get GEI."

I couldn't believe that these two guys were going to be released back into society soon. They were two scary motherfuckers. We finally reached Las Lomas, and everyone went their separate way. But I had gained a whole new perception of Brad and Aaron.

There were many other interesting characters. Adam was a cholo. We all used to go shopping in those big, white vans. I hated those vans. When we got out together, it was like *One Flew Over the Cuckoo's Nest,* and I felt like everybody knew we were the crazy nuts from the rehab. It was embarrassing. For me, anyway. Most of the guys didn't give a shit what other people thought of them. I envied them for that.

While we were on one of our shopping excursions, Adam got arrested for shoplifting. He stole a fucking bag of jelly beans and a can of smoked oysters. The next morning, he was about to get kicked out, and he didn't seem to care. He smiled and said, "I was shopping without money." That was his term for shoplifting—shopping without money. I loved it.

I don't want to forget Marcus, a very laid-back and thoughtful young Black man. His nickname was "Smurf." I had to ask why, and he told me that "Smurf" was a nickname for someone who visited a bunch of different drug stores to buy cold medicine for its pseudoephedrine, which is the main ingredient for making crystal meth. There was a limit on how much you could buy at a time; there still is. They were the small fries of the meth industry—hence, they were Smurfs.

Finally, there were two Vietnam vets, who were next-door neighbors living in studios on the first floor. Chuck and Dwight were both schizophrenics who had been living at Las Lomas for over a year. Dwight always wore a T-shirt with a big American flag emblazoned with the slogan, "THESE COLORS DON'T RUN." There was a staff member from Panama, Ernesto, who was usually a nice guy, but he always gave Dwight shit about his T-shirt. "You guys ran," he'd say. "The U.S. ran the hell out of Vietnam. And Korea, too. And if you go to Iraq, you're going to run away from there."

That kind of talk pissed off Chuck and Dwight, especially Dwight. It pissed me off, too, but I never defended them. These guys had gone through hell and came back to a country that dishonored and ignored them. I should have stood up for them; they were the ultimate wounded warriors. But I was too much of a coward to do right by them.

CHAPTER 35

Group Therapy

It was Friday morning, and I'd been out of the intensive care unit since Wednesday. Once again, I'd mixed my psych meds with a fifth of vodka and several beers and wound up back in the ICU, tethered to a ventilator. To my mind, it wasn't technically a suicide attempt; it was just another case of let's do this and see what happens.

Since I came off the ventilator and arrived in the psych ward, I'd endured the typical, albeit extremely uncomfortable, symptoms of alcohol detox. For the last few days, my mind was short-circuiting, assaulted with crazy dreams and hallucinations. My heart raced so fast I expected it to burst, and my body seesawed between drenching sweats and severe chills. But by the third day, the worst pangs of withdrawal were beginning to fade.

I was getting two milligrams of Ativan every four hours; I could have used more. I wished they still gave detox patients Librium or Valium. They worked so much better, but someone must have decided that they packed too big a punch, so instead you got Ativan. Ativan sucked.

There was no chance that I would be released until after the weekend. Weekends were boring. Most of the staff was off, and there were few groups or activities to attend. I liked the groups;

they helped pass the time. But I knew I needed to rest and let my body recuperate from the ravages of my latest binge. A fifth of vodka and a twelve-pack of beer had been my typical daily intake for the past three weeks. My body was battered—my psyche as well.

For the most part, I stayed in my room, wishing that I had the kind of one-way mirror that the TV cops used when interrogating suspects. From the safety of my room, the entire floor was a circus and entertaining to view.

I was sleepy, but it was almost time for the 9:00 check-in meeting. A patient had a better chance of being released early if he attended and participated in the therapy and meetings. The previous day, I was too wonky, but that morning I was strong enough to take a shower. After that, I headed to the meeting.

As we filed slowly into the meeting room, I noticed that my favorite fellow patient, Steven, had chosen to honor us with his presence. Steven spent most of his time patrolling the halls of our ward, making pronouncements in a surprisingly rich, baritone voice that resonated with a strong, deep timbre. I would have bet that he probably once had a career as a voice-over talent, or maybe a news announcer. That was how I liked to imagine him before, as with the rest of us, his life veered so irretrievably off course.

Steven was a handsome man, probably in his mid-sixties, with a tangled mop of curly white hair and a full white beard that needed a trim. He had been admitted days earlier, most likely petitioned for his own safety. This was my third day on the ward, and I had never seen him in anything but hospital-issue blue scrubs. Despite his wild appearance, his scrubs were always clean, and his hygiene was good. He was never dirty, and he never smelled bad.

Most patients were annoyed by his behavior and constant proclamations. Some even told him to shut up, but I found his remarks clever, even when they were nonsensical. When a patient approached him and asked why he spoke so loudly, his booming reply was, "If I don't speak in a very loud voice, I stutter." I sensed he was telling the truth.

Steven's announcements, when he was on a roll, were mesmerizing. I wanted to learn his story, but I felt too jumpy to engage him. I heard him claim that in 1975, he'd had a computer microchip implanted in his brain. I was half inclined to believe him. He was a very strange man.

As we filed slowly into the meeting room, I took a seat next to him. Including Steven and me, there were ten patients. Most were barely conscious, and a handful were about to nod off. Three others straggled in, and we numbered thirteen.

James, a tall, muscular Black man, was the psych tech in charge of the morning's meeting. He was very personable and liked to joke with the patients, but never in a mean way. I liked him.

James passed out paper and a pencil to each of us and told us to rate our anxiety and depression on a scale from one to ten. There was also a section where we were asked to note any suicidal or homicidal thoughts, also on a scale of one to ten. We then listed our goals for the day. For some people, the goal may have been as simple as taking a shower or attending groups. At the end of the day, we would meet again to report on how things had gone and whether we had reached our goals.

When everyone had completed their forms, James asked for volunteers to share what they had written. When no one volunteered, James asked Steven to begin.

Not one to follow rules, Steven had written nothing on his sheet. Nevertheless, he launched into a disjointed, thoroughly whimsical enumeration, delivered as if he were reading us newspaper headlines:

George Clooney voted most handsome man in America. Details to follow.

Ten thousand bottles of Wild Turkey delivered to Ankara.

The world awaits the news of who will become the ten-millionth and first registered nurse.

Satan makes plans to burn down Knott's Berry Farm.

James was amused. So was I, but I doubted that any of my sleepy comrades would make the connection between the whiskey and the capital of Turkey. But I gotta say, it cracked me up.

"Thank you for sharing, Steven," James said. "But you haven't told us how you are feeling this morning. Did you sleep well? What is your goal for the day? Any plans?"

"Why, thank you very much," Steven responded. Then he took a wild detour. "I have an IQ of 185, but I am very mean. I was even mean as a child. When my mother tried to breastfeed me, I would bite her nipples very hard. She threw me in the trash can 27 times."

I bit my lip. God, this guy was a treasure.

Wanting to laugh, but knowing better, James said, "Thank you, Steven. Why don't we move on? Who would like to go next? How about you, Alyssa? Would you like to share?"

Alyssa was probably in her mid-thirties, but she looked older. Because of the several thin lines surrounding her lips, I surmised she was a smoker. Her mousy brown hair hung limply to her shoulders. She twirled it nervously and cleared her throat.

"I'm Alyssa, and my anxiety level is ten. So is my depression. My suicide thoughts are an eight, and I have no thoughts of hurting anyone else. Last night I slept for six hours straight, and it was the first time in five months that I didn't have any nightmares about my boyfriend."

I learned later that Alyssa was upside-down on her mortgage

and had not made a payment since her boyfriend's suicide. Someone asked her about her boyfriend. Alyssa frowned.

James interrupted. "Alyssa, you don't need to say anything about your boyfriend."

"That's okay, I'll tell you what happened. Five months ago, my boyfriend pointed a .357 Magnum in my face and pulled the trigger. For some reason, the gun didn't go off. Then he put the gun to his head and blew his brains all over the living room. I had to get one of those crime-scene cleaning companies to clean up the . . . um . . . blood and stuff."

Someone asked, "And you're still living there? Why?"

Idiot, I thought.

"Because I own the house and have nowhere else to go."

Everyone was quiet, and the silence was excruciating. I decided to go next.

"My name is Rob. My anxiety and depression are both ten. I have no suicidal thoughts."

That wasn't exactly true, but admitting to suicidal thoughts bought you a longer stay at the hospital.

I continued. "I have no thoughts of harming anyone. I slept about six hours off and on. My goal is to attend every meeting and try to be positive, except when I talk about A.A."

I was surprised when Mary let out a laugh.

James asked, "Mary, would you like to go next?"

She was still laughing when she answered that she would.

"Oooh boy! My name is Mary. My anxiety is two, depression five. Got maybe an hour of sleep. Not suicidal, not homicidal. My goal is to try to come out of my shell. Thanks for saying that about A.A., Robert. It's like you read my mind. I hate A.A. too. I've had two sponsors, and they both fired me because they said that I was addicted to psych meds. They were the ones who were addicted.

Addicted to A.A.

"One sponsor had the nerve to tell me, 'If you choose to take psych meds, then you're not truly in recovery.'

"'Choose to take psych meds? Hunh? You think I choose to take psych meds?'

"Then she said, 'If you're taking psych meds, you shouldn't even bother celebrating your sobriety anniversary.'

"The fucking bitch. She said, 'psych meds equal no sobriety.'

"I told her, 'If I weren't taking psych meds, you would be the first person I'd kill.'"

Steven saw his opportunity and ran with it.

"She's drunk and on drugs, and uncooperative. I'll call security."

That floored me. I hadn't felt so good in a very long time.

CHAPTER 36

Psych Ward Society

Another time that Pat obtained an order for a three-day psych stay, I was, once again, an involuntary guest in the psychiatric ward of Saint Mary's Hospital. During this visit, I witnessed several examples of the human condition gone awry.

One noteworthy patient was Bernard. My room was next to his, but we didn't know one another. What happened with Bernard was that one night—more accurately, it was two in the morning—he decided to do his laundry. According to hospital policy, staff was in charge of the patients' laundry, and there was a sign-up sheet and a schedule to adhere to. This schedule was not convenient for Bernard, so he deposited his clothes in his bathroom toilet, poured in some shampoo, and commenced to flushing until his things were sufficiently clean. The problem was, of course, that a toilet is a poor substitute for a washing machine, and it overflowed. The water flooded not only the bathroom but most of Bernard's room and much of the hallway. I awoke to the panicked voices of the psych techs as they tried to stop the flow of toilet water. I turned on a light and watched as a stream of water made its way toward my room. I protected the entrance with a pile of bath towels.

The staff called housekeeping, and a custodian arrived with a bucket and mop. The toilet had finally stopped overflowing, but

Bernard's room—and much of the hall—was a swamp. Bernard, who protested that he had done nothing wrong, was escorted to the recreation room and told to stay there until the situation was under control.

I couldn't get back to sleep, so I made my way to the rec room, where I happened upon Bernard.

"Hey," I said, "looks like Lake Michigan in the hallway."

"Yeah," he said. "I needed some clean clothes. Everything I have is dirty, and the sign-up sheet for the laundry was too long. I don't know why the staff is so mad at me."

"They'll get over it," I said.

The next day, another bizarre incident occurred. Pat had dropped off two bags of things for me, mostly clothing. Visiting hours had not yet begun, so she left the bags with Lois, the head nurse. Lois took the bags from Pat but was very busy and left them on the counter, unattended. She didn't even tell me that they had been delivered.

I was waiting in line for my dinner tray and had ordered a cheeseburger and fries. The food at the hospital was not half bad. I sat with my friend, Dana, a meth addict who suffered from bipolar depression. Her face, arms, and hands were riddled with scabs that she picked at constantly and that never healed. She also had a full set of dentures that she received after losing most of her teeth in a beat-down she received at the hands of two cholas in a city park frequented by homeless people, drug dealers, and various other ne'er-do-wells. The first time I saw Dana without her dentures, I was blown away. She looked like an old crone from a fairy tale. Dana was probably in her mid-thirties, but without her dentures, she could have qualified for senior citizen discounts.

We were joined by Tammy, whom I felt sorry for. Tammy was developmentally disabled and suffered from severe unipolar depression. She received electroconvulsive therapy—it used to be called electroshock therapy—three times a week. Tammy, who also suffered from type 1 diabetes, received insulin and was on a strict diet to regulate her blood sugar. I used to order ice cream and chocolate pudding, which I would give to her. I knew that she was being monitored closely, but I wanted her to have something to enjoy in her sad and dreary life.

Brenda also ate with us. When she first arrived, she and Dana were at each other's throats, but they ironed out their differences and were civil to one another. I liked Brenda. She was crude, but she was very kind to Tammy.

Then, there was Darryl, who was a friend of Dana and was pretty rough around the edges. I think that Darryl wanted to be more than a friend to Dana. I was a bit intimidated by him, but I enjoyed his salty sense of humor. He liked to say that the hospital staff were "just patients with keys to the place."

One day, Tammy asked Darryl what he did for a living, and he said, "Well, I'm a short-order fry cook, but in my spare time, I do brain surgery." Tammy didn't get the joke.

Darryl had a favorite saying, which came in handy when living in a ward full of delusional patients. He'd say, "You lie to your friends and I'll lie to mine. Let's not lie to each other." It reminded me of something Will Rogers might have said, but it turns out they were lyrics written by an indie band with the uncanny name Guided by Voices.

So, about those bags. We were enjoying our dinner when a very large woman, whom I'd never seen before, walked past our table wearing a forest green T-shirt adorned with an embroidered, red Canadian maple leaf insignia. I recognized that shirt immediately. About seven years earlier, in September of 1998, when Pat and I were honeymooning in Whistler, British Columbia, I'd purchased that shirt along with the same version in navy blue. Those two shirts were among my favorites and were very dear to me.

"What the fuck," I said as I rose abruptly from my seat. "That's my fucking T-shirt. She's wearing my fucking T-shirt."

My dinner mates looked confused as I rushed toward the woman. I was not exaggerating when I said she was large. I was five feet eleven, and she towered over me by a good four or five inches. She was tall, sturdy, and likely weighed around 250 pounds. I was glad I had some Ativan in me because I was intimidated by her size, and I was extremely nervous.

I tried to calm myself as I said to her, "Hey, that's my shirt. What are you doing wearing my shirt? I bought that on my honeymoon. How in the hell did you get it?"

My voice was starting to shake. Lois noticed the commotion and rushed to where this very large woman and I were standing.

"What's going on here?" Lois asked.

"She's wearing my T-shirt. I bought that shirt on my honeymoon in Canada. How did you get it?" I demanded to know.

The woman answered in a calm, almost detached voice. "It's my shirt. I bought it at the mall."

"You fucking liar," I screamed. I was losing it, and I turned to Lois. "How did she get my shirt? Did my wife drop it off? Why didn't anyone tell me? What else did Pat drop off?"

"Okay, first of all, Robert, you need to calm down," Lois said.

"She stole my fucking shirt. What the hell else did she steal? What's going on?"

"Well," Lois said, "your wife did drop off two bags at the nurses' station. I was very busy, and I may have left the bags on the counter."

"You may have?" I asked. "Where are they now?"

"Let's go to the nurses' station and clear this up," she said.

The large woman who was wearing my shirt said nothing as we walked toward the station. There were no bags on the counter.

"Well, Lois, where's my stuff?" I asked.

She turned to my nemesis and asked, "Alice, what do you know about two brown paper bags that were on the counter a few minutes ago?"

"I didn't see any bags," Alice replied. "This is my shirt. I bought it at the mall." That was her story, and she was sticking to it.

We headed down a hallway to Alice's room. Coincidentally, her room was kitty-corner from mine. Lois told Alice that the two of them were going to take a quick look inside. She told me to wait in the hall, but I stayed in the doorway and could see two bags sitting on top of a dresser. I also spotted a half-empty, twenty-ounce bottle of Vanilla Coke and several empty bottles that lay on the floor. Pat had told me that she was going to bring me a six-pack of Coke, so I knew immediately that those empty bottles belonged to me.

"Those are my Vanilla Cokes," I protested. "My wife told me she was going to drop them off for me."

Lois said, "Calm down, Robert." She grabbed one of the bags and carried it to the door. She placed it on the floor and went back inside to retrieve the other bag.

"Alice, please come out and talk to Robert," she said.

Alice hesitated, but she walked to her doorway to join us. Sitting on top of one of the bags was a copy of *The Confessions of Saint Augustine*. On the cover was a depiction of Saint Augustine and his mother, Saint Monica. They were bathed in light and looking upwards, probably towards heaven. Saint Monica was cradling one of Saint Augustine's hands with both of hers.

"That book is mine," I said. "It's *The Confessions of Saint Augustine*."

"No, it's not yours," Alice said. "That's my book. See, it even has a picture of Saint Augustine. That's her on the cover."

"That's not Saint Augustine," I said. "That's St. Augustine's mother, Saint Monica. Saint Augustine was a man."

"No," she insisted, "That woman is St. Augustine."

"Wow," I said. "And where did you get all those Vanilla Cokes?" I asked her. "And how could you possibly drink them so fast?" She had to have drunk all of that soda in less than half an hour.

"Yes," Lois said, "I saw those bags at the nurses' station not more than thirty minutes ago. Did you drink all of those sodas?"

"I was thirsty," Alice said. "And they were mine anyway."

I was starting to calm down a bit. It looked like I was going to get my things back, or at least find out what had happened to them.

Lois began removing various items from the bags. One of the first things she pulled out was my blue Canada T-shirt. I was relieved to see it. The rest of the bag held more clothes from home.

"Okay then," Lois said, "all of these things look to be Robert's. Alice, I'm going to need you to go into your room and change out of the T-shirt you're wearing."

Alice was fuming, but she did as she was told. She went into her room, closed the door, and returned wearing a Hello Kitty T-shirt. She handed my shirt to Lois, who gave it to me.

"Is there anything you'd like to say to Robert?" Lois asked, expecting an apology.

"You can have the rest of the soda. There's still half a bottle left."

Wow, I thought. *Does she think I want to finish that bottle of Coke? She's fucking gross.*

"No, you keep it," I said. "I don't want it."

"Would you like to apologize to Robert for taking his things and drinking all of his soda?" Lois asked her. Alice didn't respond.

"Well, I'm going to put away my things and finish my dinner," I said.

"Good idea, Robert," Lois said. "Alice, why don't you go get your dinner tray?"

Alice released a loud belch. "I'm too full from all the soda," she said. "I don't want any dinner."

I put the bags in my room and returned to the cafeteria. Everyone was finished with their meals, but my friends had stayed to find out what was going on between Alice and me. I gave them a quick summary and began to eat my cold cheeseburger. My stomach was in knots, and I wasn't hungry anymore. After eating half my dinner, I returned to my room to put my things away and settled down to read some St. Augustine. Perhaps I could learn about acceptance and forgiveness. I calmed down and wasn't angry at Alice anymore. She probably had way more shit going on than I did. I was just glad I wasn't in her shoes.

There were many other patients at Saint Mary's who, like Alice, were right where they belonged. One was Tiffany, a young woman who was probably in her early twenties. One night, I was sitting in the rec room watching some dumb TV show with a handful of other patients when I had my encounter with Tiffany. She was dressed in pink pajama bottoms and a gauzy white blouse decorated with blue, purple, and pink flowers. The top was a few sizes too large and gave it a sort of flowing effect. She was a young, blonde girl, very short and quite plump. Her face was not unpleasant, but her weight was probably unhealthy.

As I watched television, Tiffany came skipping into the room. She made a beeline for me. God knows why; I sure didn't want the attention. She stood between me and the TV and spoke in a singsong, childlike voice.

"Hi," she said, "I'm Tiffany, what's your name?"

I was very nervous, both because of the alcohol withdrawal and the fact that all eyes were on Tiffany and me.

"Hi, Tiffany," I said. "My name is Robert, but you can call me Rob."

"I like Robert better. I'm going to call you Robert."

"That's fine by me," I told her. "What can I do for you, Tiffany?" I asked.

"Well, Robert, you're very lucky to meet me. I can do magic. In fact, if I had been allowed to keep my beautiful pearl collection, I could have turned you into a dolphin."

"A dolphin. How would you do that?" I asked.

"Well," she said, "people's heads have a very small latch hidden below the back of their ear. Right-handed people have it behind their left ear, and left-handed people have it behind their right ear. It's very hard to find. Even doctors don't know where it is. I learned this from an old woman who had amazing, magical powers. She wasn't a witch; she was much more powerful than a witch, and she didn't practice any of the black arts. She was a very good person. She died a few years ago. I'm still sad about that; I miss her.

"Anyhow, if I had one of my pearls, I could unlatch the top of your head and drop one inside. That way, whenever you went into the water, even if you were just taking a bath, you could turn yourself into a glorious dolphin. That is, if you wanted to become a dolphin. You only turn into a dolphin if you truly want to. You could go to the Pacific Ocean, and you could turn yourself into a dolphin and swim as far and as fast as you wanted. And when you were ready to become a human being again, you could just will yourself to change back."

"That sounds amazing, Tiffany. I'm sorry you don't have your jewels with you."

"Pearls," she corrected me. "Not just any old jewels. Pearls," she said. "If you ever want to become a dolphin, you can give me your phone number, and I'll call you when we get out. It will be fabulous. You'll absolutely love it."

"The thing is," I said, "I don't have a telephone. I don't even know where I'm going to be living when I get out of here."

"Well," she said, "I hope we can stay in touch. You would love being a dolphin."

"Who wouldn't?" I asked.

She yawned. "It's past my bedtime," she said. "I'm going to my room. I hope you'll consider what we talked about."

"I sure will," I said. "Good night, Tiffany.

She turned and danced off. I was relieved to see her go.

"So, Tiffany's gonna turn you into a dolphin," some tough-looking guy said.

"Looks like," I answered.

"Yeah, she tried that shit on me. I told her to fuck off."

Crude, but effective, I thought.

This guy, Carlos, was probably in his early forties. He was lean, wiry, and all tatted up. He was scary-looking, to say the least. I remember the first time I saw him. Several patients were sitting in a meeting room, waiting for the therapist to arrive for our 9:00 a.m. group, when Carlos walked to a large whiteboard in the front of the room. He grabbed a black marker and wrote: "The rapist."

Clever wordplay, I thought.

"Don't let these asshole doctors and nurses fool you," he said. "They're all a bunch of rapists and all they want to do is fuck you in the head."

Carlos made me nervous. I nodded my head after he spoke of his encounter with Tiffany. I did not doubt that he had told Tiffany to fuck off. I stood up and said goodnight. I'd had enough of these people. Creepy and crazy, that's what they were. I missed being safe at home with Pat.

I entered my room and prepared to turn in for the night. Most rooms had two beds, both of which were almost always occupied. For the time being, though, I didn't have a roommate. I loved having my own room and relished my privacy.

Another interesting patient at Saint Mary's was a woman who used to be a nurse at a Tucson hospital. Amanda had more than fifteen years of experience, but she was in the middle of a nasty divorce and had taken to drinking after her shifts. It didn't take long before she was going to work with the shakes. She needed alcohol to function. I could certainly relate to that.

Amanda decided that her only recourse was to have a few drinks before work. Of course, she chose vodka for its unsubstantiated reputation as an odorless liquor. For a while, Amanda was successful at hiding her drinking, but it didn't take long before her body demanded more than an eye-opening couple of drinks. She began to hide a pint of vodka in her purse and take a few nips throughout her workday. Soon, Amanda's body demanded alcohol at increasingly shorter intervals and, as her drinking got worse, she was failing at her job. To cut down on the alcohol, Amanda began stealing tranquilizers from the hospital.

Finally, Amanda's castle of sand was swept out to sea. She had entered an unoccupied patient's room and curled up in bed for what she told herself would be a quick nap.

Shortly after noon, the head nurse and an assistant were jostling Amanda out of her narcosis. Not only was she busted for being drunk on duty, but the staff was on to her pilfering meds. Amanda fessed up to the charges against her. She was allowed to enter a four-week treatment center and enroll in a months-long outpatient program before she would be allowed back to work.

Sadly, at the end of her four-week stay, Amanda could not beat her craving for alcohol, and she tendered her resignation. One night, about three months later, Amanda got drunk and slit her wrists. Fortunately, a friend arrived to check on her and called an ambulance that saved her life. After so many years providing help to patients, the one-time nurse was confined to a psych ward just like the rest of us. I felt bad for her, but none of the patients at Saint Mary's arrived there on a high note. Amanda clung to her vision of coping with her mental health issues, learning to live without alcohol, and having her nursing license reinstated. That was going to be one hell of a struggle.

And then there was Gina. Of all the psych patients I have ever met, Gina is the most remarkable. I met her late on a Sunday morning. I was in the rec room on a tattered old couch, seated next to Christine, an attractive young woman most likely in her early twenties. We were working on the *New York Times* crossword puzzle, and we were struggling. I have to admit that Christine, while quite fetching, was not exactly a wordsmith. She was quickly losing interest in our endeavor. I, on the other hand, was doing my best to complete the puzzle.

Gina was sitting near us on an overstuffed gray recliner. She was a petite and pretty young woman, probably in her mid to late twenties. She wore her auburn hair in a short bob and was dressed in a pair of baggy blue jeans and an oversized, olive-green, ribbed wool sweater.

She took an interest in our effort. "Do you guys mind if I join you?" she asked.

"No," I said, "we can use all the help we can get."

"Yeah," said Christine, "you can take my place. This is getting real old. I'll catch you guys later." She stood up and walked out of the rec room. Gina took a place on the couch, maintaining a healthy distance between us.

"Hi," I said, "I'm Rob. I'm not very good at the Sunday puzzle."

"I'm Gina," she said. "You're not doing half bad. You know, I've been here for almost a month, and you're the first person I've come across who has demonstrated so much as a speck of intelligence."

I blushed but managed to thank her. "I'm getting lucky with a lot of these words," I said.

"Let's work together," she said. "I bet we can knock this out in no time."

Gina was incredible. She knew the answer to every clue. After about twenty minutes, we had finished the entire crossword.

"Wow," I said, "I've never been able to finish a Sunday Times crossword, and here you zip through it in no time at all."

"Yeah," she said, "I'm pretty smart. Smart and crazy as hell. Why are you here?" she asked.

"Same old story. Drinking and mixing my meds," I said

"Oh yeah? What meds are you on?"

"Well, I take Klonopin and Vistaril for anxiety, Prozac and Remeron for depression, and Seroquel for mood disorder. Oh yeah, I take propranolol for essential tremors. You know, *Shakiest Gun in the West*; Don Knotts. Sorry, that's a movie from the late sixties; a little before your time. Anyway, I take a lot of meds."

"I appreciate your honesty. I'm on some heavy-duty meds myself. I had a very rough childhood, and that is a major understatement." She sighed deeply.

"You know what," she said, "I am an extremely introverted person. In all the days I've been here, you are the first person I've initiated a conversation with. I get hospitalized often, and I have a strict policy of keeping to myself. If someone talks to me, I'm polite, but I don't go to psych hospitals looking to make friends. I see a lot of patients exchange phone numbers before they're discharged, but I never do that. I know that I will never call anybody when I leave the hospital, so why bother? But there's something that made me want to talk with you. Could be the fact that you were working on the Sunday Times crossword. I can't tolerate stupid people, but I was interested in the crossword, and your partner didn't seem all that into it. Are the two of you close?"

"No," I said. "I just met her. She was the one who had the puzzle, and she asked if I wanted to join her. I was really glad when you showed an interest. I honestly don't think that she and I had the brainpower to solve the puzzle. But you sure did."

"You know, I have a lot of things wrong with me. I know that I'm severely mentally ill, but I also know that I'm smarter than the average bear. I don't talk much to most people, except some doctors and my regular psychiatrist. I have had the same psychiatrist since I was twenty-one. I'm twenty-eight now. I guess the doctors here could tell how fucked up I am, so I'm allowed to leave here to see my doctor. She's getting up in years and will be retiring soon, but she made me a promise that she will keep seeing me until she is either dead or incapacitated. I am so lucky to have found her. I've come a long way since I first started seeing her."

"I'm glad you found someone who can help you," I said.

"Yeah. She's the best. So easy to talk to and tell stuff. You know, it's not like you and I are going to be permanent friends—what I told you about not swapping phone numbers goes for everyone, including you—but as long as we're sitting in the same psych ward, I'll tell you a bit about myself. Thanks to my doctor, I've been able to recall a lot of shit that happened when I was barely a toddler. When I was four, I was removed from my parents' custody and eventually granted a permanent restraining order against them. They have not been allowed to see me since, and they will never have any contact with me ever again.

"After I was taken away from my parents, I wound up living in a bunch of different group homes with a ton of other screwed-up kids. That's where I learned about cutting. The doctors call it 'self-harm.' By the time I turned eleven, I was using razor blades to cut my arms and legs, and when I reached thirteen, I started cutting deeper on my torso.

"Do you still cut yourself?" I asked.

"I'm not gonna lie. Yes, I still cut myself. I don't know if I'll ever quit. I get a sort of relief when I do it. As long as I'm in the mood to reveal some of my secrets, I'll share another one. Have you ever heard of synesthesia?"

"No," I said, "I've never heard of it."

"Well, it's a term that covers a wide range, but for me—I'm what's called a synesthete—synesthesia comes in a form where certain words or letters have a color and, sometimes, an odor to them. Like, let's say, for me, the letter 'A' is a glimmering gold, like a bright sunrise, and a 'B' is crimson red. And words. Certain words bring on powerful sensations. For instance, the word 'home' is imbued with a dark, misty gray that smells strongly of musk."

"This is probably a strange question, but are there any aspects of your synesthesia that you enjoy?" I asked her.

"Well, I don't know if I can say I like the effects, but I'm pretty used to them, and I don't mind them. Okay, Rob, I've been saving the best news for last. Let me ask you, have you ever met anyone who has dissociative identity disorder?"

"No," I said, "I know a little about bipolar depression and mood swings, but I don't think that's what you're referring to."

"Oh, no, it's a lot different than bipolar mood swings. I have three distinct personalities. There's me, Gina, and then there's a little girl who's four years old and very smart; she is the one who remembers my early childhood most clearly. She's also very . . . let's say snotty. She's a snotty little brat. Her name is Sofia. She generally manifests herself when I'm choosing what to wear at the start of the day. She strongly prefers colorful clothes, and she hates my baggy attire. She wants me to wear better-fitting clothes, and she throws temper tantrums when I don't do what she wants."

"Does she ever visit you here in the hospital?" I asked.

She laughed. "Absolutely. Every morning after I take a shower, and any time I change my clothes. Little Miss Sofia doesn't miss a beat. She's always showing up to suggest—or should I say, demand—which outfits she wants me to wear. She can be extremely annoying, but other than the whining and the hissy fits, she's pretty harmless. Sometimes, I even enjoy her company; she can be pretty sweet when she wants to. She has told my doctor and me so many things that I don't remember, and when she describes specific incidents, she doesn't get emotional. In fact, she is remarkably detached when relating even the most godawful episodes of my childhood."

"And your third personality, who is that?" I asked.

"My third personality is a charming little Russian Blue, female cat with the most piercing, bright green eyes."

"What happens when you become a cat? What's it like? Does this cat know that you're human?" I asked.

She laughed again. "Lots of questions, Rob. I guess I can understand your difficulty imagining me as a cat. Ernestine—that's her name—shows up regularly when I wake up in the morning and when I go to bed each night. She's very loving and affectionate, and she helps me muster the courage to face each new day. She also helps me unwind in the evening. No matter how bad a day I've had, Ernestine knows how to smooth me out. She is such a reliable companion. She encourages me to settle down and relax. And she is extremely patient. I love my Ernestine; she's the best."

"Does Ernestine talk—I mean, like a human? Does she speak English?"

"No, Ernestine doesn't speak English or any other human language. She communicates with a wide variety of meows and a soothing assortment of purrs and trills. She's a true friend, and she's an amazingly calming influence on me, unlike little Sofia. So, Rob, what do you think of the Gina I've revealed to you?"

"Well, first of all, Gina, I feel honored that you chose to trust me with your story. I am also sorry beyond words that you had to grow up the way you did, and I'm glad you've found a great doctor whom you can trust."

"Unconditionally," she said, "I trust her unconditionally."

"Yes," I said, "unconditionally. That's beautiful."

She rose slowly from the couch. "I'm feeling sleepy, so I'm going to take a nap. Thank you for listening to me, not judging me. You're a good person, Rob."

"Thank you for talking with me," I said. "Enjoy your nap."

She smiled as she walked away. I hoped that one day she might find a modicum of peace.

CHAPTER 37

Telemedicine

On a June morning in 2010, I checked in at the AYUDA Behavioral Health Center for an appointment with Dr. Rebecca Harris, a psychiatrist whom I had never met before. Pat and my AYUDA case manager, Carla Delarosa, were with me.

As we were seated in her office, Dr. Harris looked up from her computer and said, "Apparently, you're being prescribed a total of six milligrams of clonazepam per day. That is far too high a dose. You should not be taking more than four milligrams a day, and even that should eventually be discontinued. Clonazepam is not a drug we encourage our clients to take. In fact, I am not comfortable with prescribing any benzodiazepines whatsoever."

I got upset and told her that I had been taking that dose of clonazepam for years and that lowering it was a huge mistake. She waved me off and said that she did not appreciate being told her business. That really pissed me off.

"You don't know me," I said. "I don't think you even know what you're doing."

"How dare you talk to me like that? I am a medical professional, and as of now, I am discontinuing your clonazepam."

"You stupid fucking bitch," I screamed. "You don't have a fucking clue."

Her face went crimson.

"I want you out of my office right now. No one talks to me like that. Go see Dr. Hamid or someone else. We're through here."

"What if Dr. Hamid can't see him?" asked Carla.

"I don't care what happens to him. No patient is going to treat me with that level of disrespect."

I jumped up and said, "Fuck you, you fucking ignoramus."

Carla and Pat each grabbed one of my elbows.

"Rob," Pat said, "let's go. This isn't doing any good."

Pat and Carla yanked me out of the small office. As we stood in the hallway, I told them that I absolutely could not function without my Klonopin. We walked to the lobby, and Carla told us to wait. She went into the main office to talk to someone.

"Rob," Pat said, "you can't talk to these people like that. They have way more power than you do."

"Pat," I said, "you know I can't lose my Klonopin."

"I know. We'll do something, but you can't call her names like that."

"I'm sorry," I said. "She was just such a self-righteous bitch."

Pat said nothing. She was exasperated.

After about ten minutes, Carla came out to the lobby. My therapist, Elizabeth, was with her.

"Robert," Carla said, "we're going to do a teleconference with a doctor in Phoenix. Let's see what he can do for you."

"And I'll be with you to back you up," said Elizabeth as she began massaging my shoulder. I bristled. I was in no mood to be touched.

"Follow me," Carla said, "we're ready for the teleconference."

"Remember, Robert, keep your cool," Elizabeth said.

Pat and I entered a small office, accompanied by Carla and Elizabeth. There was a television attached high on the wall. We each took a seat facing the screen. Carla had a remote control. She pointed it toward the TV and clicked it.

We were now watching a screen occupied by a man with thinning gray hair and a pair of thick glasses.

"That's Dr. Randolph," Carla said. "He's agreed to speak with you."

"But . . . wait," I said, "he knows nothing about me or my case."

"This is the best we could do," she said. "Give him a chance, Robert."

"Okay," I said. What else could I do?

"Hello, Dr. Randolph, I'm Carla Delarosa, case manager for the client, Robert Rickelman. And this is Robert." She gestured toward me.

"His wife Patricia is here, as well as his therapist, Elizabeth Hennessey."

"Hello," said the doctor. "Well, let's get started."

"Dr. Randolph," Carla said, "Robert has had a difference of opinion with one of our psychiatrists, Dr. Harris, over his dosage of clonazepam."

"And what was the difference of opinion?" the doctor asked.

"Well, Dr. Harris wanted to decrease Robert's dosage from six milligrams per day to four milligrams, and Robert is not comfortable with the cutback."

"Six milligrams? Did you say the patient is currently taking six milligrams a day? That's far too high a dose. I have to weigh in on Dr. Harris's behalf. I agree that Mr. Rickelman's dose needs to be reduced."

I stood up. "What are you talking about? I've been on this dose for six years, and it has been a lifesaver for me. How can you order such a drastic reduction without even knowing me or reading my file?"

"Excuse me. I will not be addressed in that tone by a patient. Especially a drug-seeking patient who doesn't know what's good for him."

"You're a fucking quack!" I screamed. "You don't know shit, you fucking moron."

"Robert," Carla said, "please calm down. This isn't helping."

Elizabeth was pissed. "You cannot behave like this and expect anyone to help you," she said.

"I don't care. This asshole doesn't know jack shit about me, and he wants to turn my life upside down."

"I won't stay here if you're going to act like this. He's the doctor, and you need to respect him," Elizabeth said.

"Fine, then leave me the fuck alone. You told me you wanted to help me, but you're just toeing the company line. You don't give a shit about me. And this fucking idiot doctor, he doesn't care either."

"That's it," she said, "I'm out of here."

"Fine. Go, I don't give a fuck. Get the fuck out of here."

Pat tried to calm me down. "Rob, please, this isn't helping."

"She's right, Robert, you need to calm down," Carla said. At least she wasn't selling me out like Elizabeth.

The doctor was still on the screen. Carla apologized to him for my behavior.

"I'm sorry, doctor, Robert is extremely distraught."

"I don't care how distraught he is. I'm the doctor, he's the patient. And no patient has the right to talk to me like that. As of now, I am lowering his dose of clonazepam to four milligrams. That's the end of this. I'll fax you my orders."

Before I could rattle off any more obscenities, the screen went dark.

"Well, looks like that's it," Carla said. "I'm sorry, Robert, but you really lost it."

"Oh, Rob," Pat said, "you need to calm yourself down."

"I'm sorry, but he doesn't know anything about me, and he's lowering my Klonopin from Phoenix, by a fucking teleconference. He's a useless idiot.

"Let's go out to the lobby," Carla said. "I'll check the fax and see what it says."

"Thank you," Pat said.

"Yeah, thanks, Carla," I said. "Thank you for trying."

Pat and I sat in the lobby, waiting.

"We'll figure out something, Rob," Pat said. She rubbed my arm gently.

In about twenty minutes, Carla came out and sat with Pat and me.

"I'm sorry, but I have some bad news. The doctor wrote an order decreasing your clonazepam to four milligrams."

"Son of a bitch," I said.

"There's more. He wrote in his orders that you will not be given any prescriptions. You're going to have to come in every Wednesday, and a nurse practitioner and I will fill a med box for you. You'll be doing this until someone in authority says that you can fill your own meds again."

"What do they think?" I asked. "That I'm gonna try to commit suicide? They'd probably like that."

"So," Pat asked, "when do we get this week's meds?"

Carla said, "Jason Lewis is an NP, and he's going to order your meds. You can come in on Wednesday, the day after tomorrow; he'll give you a weekly med box, and he'll fill it. I'll be there too. You'll have to come in every Wednesday until . . .well . . . let's just plan on every Wednesday until something changes."

"Thank you, Carla," Pat said. "You've been so nice and so patient.

You're the only one here who honestly cares about my husband."

"Yeah, well, I'm so sorry about how everything went down," she said.

"So, we'll see you on Wednesday?" Pat asked.

"Yes. Wednesday at 2:00. Robert, do you have enough meds until then?"

I nodded my head. I was stunned by everything that had happened.

"Okay then," Pat said. "Thanks for all of your help, Carla. We'll see you Wednesday."

"Goodbye, guys," she said. "Try to hang in there, Robert."

I stood up, feeling dizzy. "Thanks for everything, Carla. You did your best. I appreciate that," I said.

Pat and I walked out to the parking lot and got in the car. Pat insisted on driving. That was for the best.

"Wow, Rob, you really went off the rails in there."

"Can we file a complaint about this?" I asked her.

"Maybe, but it would have been better if you hadn't said all that stuff. It's not going to help your situation."

The next few weeks were brutal. The lower dose of Klonopin left me jittery and on edge. I did nothing but stay in bed or lie on the couch all day long. I didn't step outside, except for the one day each week when Pat and I would go to AYUDA to have my med box filled.

One Wednesday, Elizabeth saw me in the lobby and approached me.

"How are you doing, Rob? I've been worried about you."

I just stared at the floor until she walked away. I was through with her; she wasn't my therapist anymore.

CHAPTER 38

Gas Wars

I had been substitute teaching for the past few years. It was a shitty job, but I needed the money to supplement my monthly Social Security check. We had one more week of school until winter break, and I wanted to get my last days in. But after a quarter of a million miles, our dependable 1997 Toyota Corolla was calling it quits. Our mechanic said we were looking at $3000 or more in repairs, and the car wasn't worth fixing.

So, Pat and I rented a car at the airport on the south side of Tucson, and at the end of the week, we went to return the rental. Pat was driving our Versa, and I drove the loaner. It was 5:30 on a warm Friday evening. The gas station nearest the airport was teeming with cars. Every pump was taken, but I needed to fill up. I crept along in a slow-moving circle, looking for an opening. Finally, a car pulled away, and I made a quick U-turn to get to the pump. Just as I was about to turn into the space, a big, old, rusty blue SUV with a faded gray hood made a move for the same spot. I zipped in and got to the pump ahead of the beater.

The driver of the SUV, a large and angry woman, emerged from her vehicle. Her long, bleached-blond hair was a dirty, tangled mess, and she wore torn blue jeans and a yellow tank top that accentuated every roll of fat. Straightaway, she set about screaming and swearing. I eased out of the car and said, "Sorry, I got here first."

"Fuck you, you mother-fucking asshole," she yelled.

I tried to blow her off, but she was furious. I checked to find the gas cap, and it was on the other side of the car. *Fuck*. I had rented a Mitsubishi Eclipse, a fairly small car, and I hoped that I could stretch the hose far enough for the nozzle to reach. I unscrewed the cap and, as I walked to the pump, I heard a loud voice as a man emerged from the SUV.

"Hey, motherfucker, you just stole my wife's pump."

Oh, great, some fucking guy wanted to defend his wife's honor. I was 57 years old, paunchy, slow, and the fucking guy wanted to fight. My stomach was doing flips, and I was nervous as hell, but I had to let things play out.

I turned to face my opponent. He was pretty stout. Maybe five-foot-ten, about 200 pounds. His hands were grimy and smudged. He was wearing baggy, brown shorts and a tight black T-shirt. And he had some guns, I'll give him that. Those were some big, strong arms on him.

He was a lot younger than I was—late twenties, maybe early thirties. I knew I was fucked, but I walked toward him, trying to show a bit of swagger.

He was probably about 20 feet away, advancing toward me and looking fearsome. And, fool that I was, I continued approaching him. He said to me, "What the fuck is your fucking problem, talking shit to my wife?"

"I just said I was here first." My hands were shaking like crazy. I stuck them in my pockets. Not a good idea. I pulled them out.

"Who the fuck do you think you are, you dumb motherfucker?"

"Yeah, you stupid mother-fucking piece of shit." His wife, the chick with the big gut, big ass, and big mouth, taunted me.

I went for broke. "Shut the fuck up, you stupid fucking bitch." *Did I just say that? Whoa.*

The guy came at me quickly. I took off my glasses. I didn't want him to break them when he smashed me in the face. But I couldn't see shit, so I put them back on.

Oh my God, I thought. *Rob, you are so fucked.*

He was right in front of me. I needed to do something. I took a swing with my right fist and hit him in the neck, then quickly threw another punch. This one hit the other side of his neck. He stepped back a few paces. I didn't knock him down. I might have hurt him, but I didn't knock him down.

He smiled and said, "Man, you best be getting your ass to the gym if that's all you got. Yeah, man, you seriously need to get to the gym."

I couldn't believe he didn't take a swing at me. Pat came running.

"Rob, Rob," she pleaded. "Stop it! Stop fighting."

The guy's wife was going nuts. "You motherfucking cocksucker. You just punched my husband. I should call the fucking cops on your fucking ass."

But she didn't. She called to her man. "Come on, babe. We gotta go."

They walked to their SUV. She got in on the driver's side. As he opened his door, he said, "Damn, man, you throw some weak fucking punches. Yeah, man, get your sorry ass to the gym."

I watched nervously as they pulled into traffic. The woman unrolled her window and gave me the finger. "Fuck you, mother fucker," she shouted.

"Rob, what just happened?" Pat asked. "I can't believe he didn't hit you. He must have some outstanding warrants or something."

"Yeah," I said. So much for my fighting skills, but I knew Pat was right. That guy must have been afraid of the cops. Otherwise, I'd be lying in a pool of my own fucking blood.

"Pat, it wasn't my fault. That chick was flipping out. And the husband came out of nowhere."

To my surprise, Pat agreed. "I know. She was going nuts. That *gorda* was crazy."

Back at the pump, I maneuvered the nozzle to reach the gas door. I unkinked the hose, the gas started flowing, and I filled the tank. As I finished, two Chicanos started calling me from their big, silver Chevy pickup. They were both wearing white wife-beater T-shirts.

"Hey, bro. You did good. You gave that guy some good hits," the driver said.

"Yeah, you did good for an old guy," said his passenger.

"Thanks," I said. "I don't even know what happened."

"That fucking chick was *loca*. And you gave that dude some good blows."

I laughed. "Thanks, I thought he was going to kill me."

"No, man, you did good. You mixed it up good, *vato.*"

They had an 18-pack of Budweiser in the truck, and they were each holding a cold can. The beer looked mighty tasty.

"You take care, man," the driver said. "You're dangerous, huh?"

Then he feigned some moves toward me, like a boxer in the ring. I flinched.

"Hey, homes, I'm just goofing. You're good people, bro." Both the driver and his passenger traded fist bumps with me before they drove off.

"Thanks for the show, man. Right on, bro. You did good," they hollered to me.

Finally, with the tank full, Pat and I got into our cars and drove to the airport. My hands were still shaking.

CHAPTER 39

Anniversary Flowers

A few years after his marriage to Elise, my father was diagnosed with a very aggressive form of prostate cancer. It did not take long for the cancer to spread to his blood, bones, and skull. By the fall of 2011, my father's condition was hopeless. I visited him every Saturday and Sunday, keeping him company and trying to make up for the times when I wasn't a very good son. I think he appreciated my effort. He wrote me a letter before he died, thanking me for the time I had been spending with him.

We spent Saturday, October 29, together, which provided Elise some relief from the stress of being his primary caregiver. I arrived at 9:00 a.m., and Elise left for the gym. She returned just after 11:00, changed clothes, and left to enjoy a well-deserved afternoon of shopping at Tucson's Park Mall.

My dad and I passed the first few hours watching Jon Stewart and Stephen Colbert, but his pain was getting worse, and with it came severe nausea and a relentless bout of diarrhea. I escorted him to the bathroom several times. I felt helpless as he struggled to maintain his dignity after soiling himself in bed, but he carried himself with measured grace.

Elise returned from shopping just after 4:00. My father embraced her, then asked if she'd leave the room so he could speak with me. After she had left, my dad whispered to me with an air of embarrassment, "Rob, could you do me a big favor? I haven't even been able to get Elise an anniversary card. Would you mind going to the store and buying a card and maybe some flowers? It's our seventh anniversary."

I sensed his deep despair.

"Sure, I'll go right now."

I had no money on me, so when I stepped outside, I called Pat to ask if she would meet me to pay for the card and flowers. She said she would leave immediately for the Walgreens on Country Club and Speedway. I arrived first and began looking at cards. I found one that touched me, and right there in the Hallmark section of the store, I started bawling like a baby. I fought to stifle my sobbing, but I couldn't keep the tears from flowing.

When Pat arrived, I handed her the card, and she paid the cashier. My eyes were red; my cheeks tear-streaked and moist. I felt embarrassed, but there was no reason to be. After all, who wouldn't cry on such a sad mission? Buying an anniversary card for my sick and dying father, who did not have the strength to get out of bed?

The Walgreens didn't sell flowers, so we drove to the Whole Foods Store. I asked a clerk if we could get a dozen roses. She apologized and said that they were out of roses. We picked out a dozen beautiful red Gerbera daisies. The cashier was a Latina in her late twenties, and she was very sweet. I told her we were buying the flowers for my dying dad to give to his wife on their anniversary. She seemed genuinely touched and told us how sorry she was.

We left the store and my car, and Pat drove me to Elise and my father's house. I asked her to park where our car wouldn't be seen. I left the car and walked to their door. I placed the card and flowers out of sight, behind a large planter, and rang the bell.

When Elise answered, I asked her if I could talk to my dad in private. She looked a bit confused but said of course, and went to wait in their study.

I grabbed the card and flowers and walked to the living room, where the hospital bed faced the TV. My dad saw the flowers and smiled.

"How much were they?" he asked.

"Free," I said. "They were giving free flowers with every card."

"Please, Rob, I need to pay for them." But he remembered that he didn't have his wallet. It was in the study.

"Can I pay you tomorrow?" he asked.

"Sure, tomorrow's fine."

I gave him the flowers first.

"They're beautiful," he said. "Thank you so much, Rob. Thank you for everything."

I had a huge lump in my throat. I fought to hold back the tears.

"I have the card," I said. "Do you have a pen to sign it?"

He had one handy on a stand next to his bed. I gave him the card, and he wrote a note to Elise.

"Well, I'd better be going." I struggled to keep my composure. "I love you, Dad. I wish I could have been a better son. Not let you down, not been so selfish."

I bent to kiss his forehead, put his hands in mine, and caressed them.

"So long, Dad. Happy Anniversary."

"Thank you, Rob," he said.

I was crying pretty hard as I left the room. I went outside and walked to the car. Pat was concerned.

"If you're not up to driving, we can get the other car in the morning," she said.

"No, thanks, that's okay. I can drive."

"I'm going to follow close behind you; make sure you're okay."

We drove to my car, and Pat dropped me off. I pulled out of the parking lot into the heavy traffic of Speedway Boulevard. When we got home, I was exhausted and sad, but I knew I'd done right by my dad. Pat and I were with him and Elise when he died peacefully on January 1, 2012. We weren't always close, but I miss him. He had his faults, but he did the best he could.

CHAPTER 40

Mountain Market Liquor Store

It was a mild Thursday morning, January 10, 2013. Pat had gone to work, but her daughter, Madeline, was home. By 10:00 a.m., I was shaky, and I needed alcohol. I used to go to Ace Hardware and have copies made of the keys for our two cars, a 1996 Geo Metro and a 1997 Toyota Corolla, and I'd use the keys to the car Pat left home to drive to the liquor store.

But the game changed when we got rid of those cars and purchased a 2009 Nissan Versa and a 2011 Sentra. The keys for those cars were a new generation. Each car had two remote control key fobs, and Pat guarded them like a hawk. Back then, these remotes could only be reproduced at a Nissan dealer, and they cost over $200 apiece. I could not afford to pay that price for copies, so my days of driving to the liquor store were over.

I prepared for my walk to the store. I pulled on some jeans and a sweatshirt, grabbed a twenty from a hiding place under the mattress, and headed out of my bedroom and toward the back door. Madeline could hear me from her bedroom and came out to see what I was up to.

"Rob, what are you doing?"

"Nothing, don't worry about it," I said.

Things were a lot easier when she was younger and not yet onto me and my tricks, but she was almost 20.

I put on a pair of rubber beach sandals that were in very poor condition and headed out of the yard toward the Mountain Market Liquor Store. As I walked east toward the store, Madeline called out to me.

"Rob, what are you doing? Come back, Rob."

I ignored her and walked as fast as I could in that worn-out pair of sandals. The store was about a ten-minute walk from the house. The old flip-flops kept falling off my feet, and I had to stop each time I lost one to put it back on.

I finally reached the liquor store and went inside. I asked for two bottles of vodka, fifths, which they kept behind the counter. A middle-aged, Indian gentleman grabbed the bottles and placed them on the counter.

"That will be eighteen dollars, thirty-three cents."

My hands were shaking as I handed him the twenty. He put the bottles in a paper bag and returned a dollar and change. I stuffed the money into my pocket, grabbed the bottles, and left. I needed a drink fast, and I ducked into a parking lot that was located next to the liquor store. I took out a bottle and unscrewed the cap. I took a big draw of vodka, probably about three or four ounces, waited a minute for the burn to subside, then took another long swig.

Just then, a middle-aged guy in a suit and tie came out of an office building and yelled, "Hey, what are you doing? This is private property. I'm going to call the cops."

Suddenly, our silver Versa came whipping into the driveway with a furious-looking Pat behind the wheel. I guzzled down about five or six ounces until the booze started pouring out of my nose and mouth.

Pat screeched to a halt, jumped out of the car, and ran toward me. She grabbed the bottle, almost breaking my front teeth in the process. She poured the remaining booze onto the pavement, grabbed the unopened bottle, and smashed it into the ground. My heart sank. What a terrible waste of good booze.

At the same time, the guy from the store ran out shouting, "Hey, you! You are barred from this store. You are never allowed in here again. Don't you ever come back!"

Pat told me to get in the car. I did as I was told.

"How could you do this with Madeline at home?' Pat screamed. "What the hell is wrong with you?"

I stayed silent. I couldn't believe that I'd lost all of my vodka. Pat hit the accelerator and took off like a bat out of hell. As we pulled into our driveway, Pat said, "You need to go to the hospital. I'm calling 911."

I wanted to make a run for it, but what could I do with a dollar and a half and a broken pair of *chanclas*? I was screwed, and nothing I would say was going to change Pat's mind. I was grateful that I had managed to consume about half of the first fifth. We entered the house, and Pat dialed 911. I sat on the couch and waited.

Minutes later, I heard sirens approaching. Two cop cars arrived, and a few minutes later, a Tucson Fire Department ambulance showed up. One of the cops was a plain-looking, tall, blonde female. Then, there was a male cop who looked at me as if I were a piece of shit, and that's what I felt like.

He talked to Pat as if I weren't even there. "Depending on what the paramedics decide, we can either take him to the hospital or —"

At this point, the paramedics took over.

"Robert," one of the paramedics said, "what's going on with you? Have you been drinking?"

"Yes," I said.

"Ask him if he's taken any of his meds. He's on a lot of psych meds," Pat said.

"Robert, have you been mixing your meds with alcohol?"

I nodded.

"What meds, Robert?"

"A few Klonopins and a few Seroquels."

The vodka I'd pounded was kicking in, especially since it was consumed with the Klonopin and Seroquel. I was full-blown blotto.

The paramedic said, "Okay, Robert, since we don't know what quantities of drugs you took, and since you are very drunk, we're going to take you to the hospital."

I had been through this drill so many times that I just let things take their course. I was so hammered that I felt no guilt or shame for the hell I was putting Pat through.

The firemen helped me up from the couch and onto a stretcher. Then they tightened safety straps on me so I wouldn't fall off, and they wheeled me out to the ambulance. The paramedics told Pat that they were taking me to the Banner South Medical Center. We drove without lights or sirens. One paramedic stayed in the cabin with me, monitoring my vitals. The other one drove. Pat followed us to the hospital in the Versa.

I was taken to the ER and given a room immediately, which was one perk of coming to the hospital in an ambulance. I was making statements that indicated I was suicidal, so Pat asked the doctors to keep me for a 72-hour psych hold. I was too high to have any part in the decision, but Pat always looked out for me, no matter what.

The medical team hooked me up to an EKG, constantly checked my vitals, did blood draws, and inserted an IV needle into a vein on the top of my right hand to provide fluids and electrolytes. The bag contained thiamine and multivitamin components that gave the liquid its yellow color.The ER staff called it a "banana bag".

I had been in the ER for about four or five hours, and they had given me no medications. That made sense because I already had so much shit in my system. Pat had left—she had to work—and I drifted in and out of consciousness. I remember being very cold; ERs were always cold, probably to keep the doctors and nurses alert.

The haze started to lift a bit, and I checked the clock. It was 6:00 p.m. I was starting to feel nauseated and shaky. When a nurse came in to check on me, I asked if I could get anything for nausea and anxiety.

She said, "I'll ask the doctor to write you something for the nausea, but we need to wait before we can give you any sedatives. You were just too drunk when you came in."

At about 6:30, the nurse came to me with a syringe. "The doctor ordered some Zofran for your nausea. It's going to make you sleepy."

I missed Pat. Funny how that always happened. I would scheme and connive ways to get a drink when Pat was at work, and after she'd busted me, I'd be pissed. But after several hours in the ER, everything I'd done to Pat would sink in, and I would feel guilty and selfish. I was a fucking asshole who didn't deserve such a wonderful wife.

At midnight, I received more Zofran and two milligrams of Ativan to ease the withdrawal.

At 1:00 a.m., I was moved to the psych ER across the hall. At 6:00 a.m., I received more Zofran and Ativan. On Friday afternoon, I was moved to the psych ward. A nurse took a bag containing my street clothes and shoes and unlocked the door to an examination room.

"Please remove your gown and socks," said the nurse.

I did as she said, and a psych tech inspected me for contraband.

"He's good," said the tech.

At the same time, another tech was removing my belongings and carefully examining them for any prohibited items, most importantly, anything I could use to harm myself, such as a belt, shoelaces, or even a pencil or pen.

"Just a pair of jeans, sweatshirt, shoes, socks, and underwear," he said.

"Okay," said the no-nonsense nurse. "Put them in a locker for him."

"What size pants and shirt do you wear?" asked the nurse.

"Extra-large," I said. "Maybe double X."

She handed me a pair of blue scrub pants and a matching shirt, both extra-large. I put them on. She then gave me a beige pair of hospital socks with non-slip rubber bottoms.

"We prefer that once our patients have acclimated themselves, they wear their street clothes on the ward," she said.

"Okay," I said. "Um . . . you haven't told me your names."

The nurse, stern-looking and reed-thin, said, "My name is Barbara. This is Oscar, and this is Ralph." She gestured toward the two techs.

Barbara asked me a bunch of questions about my health and whether I was still suicidal. I answered that the thought had crossed my mind. When Barbara was finished, she told Ralph to take me to my room. My roommate was snoring loudly.

While I was in a common area, a very large, very angry, white guy got into a heated argument with a big Black guy who spoke English with a Spanish accent. The white guy's name was Adam, and he lunged at the Hispanic guy, Renaldo, who promptly punched Adam square in the nose. There was blood everywhere; I was sure his nose was broken. Thankfully, both Adam and Renaldo got kicked out, and I guessed that they were either headed to jail or some other psych hospital.

The fighting wasn't limited to the men. A handful of female patients were constantly quarreling and threatening to do bodily harm to each other. The word of the day was "Fuck." "Fuck you, fuck this, fuck off, fucking bitch, and I'm gonna fuck you up."

Saturday morning, two women in their late twenties got into an argument that resulted in face-slapping and hair-pulling. One of the women ended up with a handful of red hairs yanked from her adversary. Those two were shipped out as well.

I was in no condition to deal with the constant turmoil, so I spent most of the weekend in bed. There were no meetings or activities that Saturday or Sunday.

After Monday morning breakfast, I was summoned to a doctor's office. I was surprised to find three female psychiatrists waiting for me. I was glad to see them, but things took an unexpected turn.

"Robert," said one of the women, "I'm Dr. Whitmore, and these are my associates, Dr. Beckman and Dr. Conyer."

"I'm very glad to meet you all. I haven't talked to a doctor since I was admitted. It will be nice to get some insight from you."

"I'm sorry, Robert," Dr. Whitmore said, "but we are here to advise you that, because the nurses and techs reported no issues with you over the weekend, we are going to discharge you."

"What? When?" I asked. I was floored.

"Your discharge is effective immediately. We've drawn up your papers, and you'll be free to leave once the nurses have determined where you'll be living."

“Don’t I even get a single session? I have so many questions to ask you.”

“Well, we see that you are a patient at AYUDA, and you will be seeing one of their doctors in a day or so.”

“So that’s it. Wow. This is unbelievable.” My hands began to tremble; I was so angry.

“Okay, thanks for all your expertise and concern.” My voice was dripping with sarcasm. Nervous sarcasm.

I turned, left the office, and walked to the phone to call Pat. She was shocked to hear that I was being released, but there wasn’t anything we could do.

“I’ll come pick you up, Rob. What time should I be there?” she asked.

“Any time you can make it will be good; the sooner the better.”

I was so pissed that all I could think of was getting good and fucking drunk. I would bide my time and wait for my opportunity. In the meantime, Pat picked me up, and for the life of me, I do not know why I haven’t had a drink since January 10, 2013, the day I caused a commotion at the Mountain Market Liquor Store.

About the Author

Robert Rickelman grew up in the suburbs of Chicago. He studied at the University of Illinois and John Marshall Law School. In 1995, he moved to Tucson.

Following a suicide attempt in 1996, Robert was diagnosed as Seriously Mentally Ill (SMI). He still carries this SMI designation.

Robert earned his BA in Spanish from the University of Arizona in 2000 and has been published in various literary magazines. His story, "Phyllis," was awarded *Inscape Magazine's* 2018 Nonfiction Editors' Choice Award. He lives in Tucson with his wife, Pat, who has never given up on him.

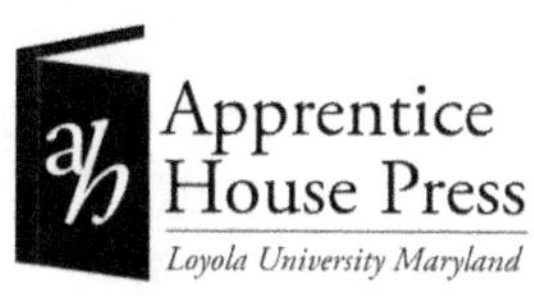

Apprentice House is the country's only campus-based, student-staffed book publishing company. Directed by professors and industry professionals, it is a nonprofit activity of the Communication & Media Department at Loyola University Maryland.

Using state-of-the-art technology and an experiential learning model of education, Apprentice House publishes books in untraditional ways. This dual responsibility as publishers and educators creates an unprecedented collaborative environment among faculty and students, while teaching tomorrow's editors, designers, and marketers.

Eclectic and provocative, Apprentice House titles intend to entertain as well as spark dialogue on a variety of topics. Financial contributions to sustain the press's work are welcomed. Contributions are tax deductible to the fullest extent allowed by the IRS.

To learn more about Apprentice House books or to obtain submission guidelines, please visit www.apprenticehouse.com.

Apprentice House Press
Communication & Media Department
Loyola University Maryland
4501 N. Charles Street
Baltimore, MD 21210
410-617-5265
info@apprenticehouse.com • www.apprenticehouse.com

www.ingramcontent.com/pod-product-compliance
Lightning Source LLC
LaVergne TN
LVHW010604100826
845148LV00014B/2845